Praise for Rolf Gates's

*Meditations on
Intention and Being*

"Rolf presents his wealth of yoga knowledge and his life experiences
in such a way that you feel encouraged to follow suit. He combines
the more complex teachings of Buddha with specific examples that
guide the reader through very meaningful and accessible chapters.
Not only does he talk the talk—he walks the walk too."
    —Kathryn Budig, yoga teacher and author of *Aim True*

"*Meditations on Intention and Being* is a wonderful balance between
personal story and traditional Eastern philosophy, and offers an inspi-
rational and informed perspective on the place of yoga, mindfulness,
and compassion in our everyday lives."   —Beryl Bender Birch,
                    author of *Power Yoga* and *Yoga for Warriors*

"Rolf has done it again. These reflections are so down-to-earth and
practical that you relax just reading them. If you are interested in living your life from the inside out, this is the book you want to start
your day with."   —Congressman Tim Ryan,
        author of *A Mindful Nation: How a Simple Practice Can Help Us
    Reduce Stress, Improve Performance, and Recapture the American Spirit*

"Inspiring and accessible. Rolf's intimate writing about his own life journey demonstrates to the reader how to apply the key teachings from yoga and mindfulness in everyday life."
—Phillip Moffitt, author of *Dancing with Life* and
Emotional Chaos to Clarity

"Gates's searching meditations on life's pains and imperfections, and the huge challenges we face in meeting those pains with compassion, are among the most eloquent I have read in modern yoga literature."
—Rob Schware, executive director, the Give Back
Yoga Foundation; president, the Yoga Service Council

"Filled with beautifully polished reflections on life and ancient wisdom teachings. Rolf's personal honesty and ability to craft a lush story make page after page a brilliant, insightful gift."
—R. Nikki Myers, founder,
Y12SR (The Yoga of 12-Step Recovery)

"A masterful work of art. My heart is more open, my mind is quieter, and my purpose is clearer after reading this extraordinary book."
—Sarah Gardner, founder, Yoga Reaches Out

"*Meditations on Intention and Being* whispers us through a heartfelt journey into both inward and outward dimensions. This book challenges the reader, but more important, supports and instills hope. I recommend it for anyone seeking to live a better, more fulfilling life."
—Matthew Sanford, president and CEO,
Mind Body Solutions; author of *Waking*

"*Meditations on Intention and Being* is a gift of Rolf's accessible and uncanny wisdom that we can enjoy from our favorite chair, sofa, or yoga mat right at home." —Brian Leaf, author of *Misadventures of a Garden State Yogi*

"An excellent guide to further all of us down our personal path of knowledge and understanding. As Rolf talks about how some of these life lessons came to him, we see how they often appear in simple, everyday occurrences. As he points out, we should take these teachings where we find them and apply them however works. So no matter what happens, no matter where we find ourselves in the metaphorical sense, just keep paddling." —Gerry Lopez, legendary surfer, actor, and author of *Surf Is Where You Find It*

"Rolf speaks to us out of his own struggles and learnings, his own ongoing path of growth, and his own authenticity, humility, and self-compassion." —Gordon Wheeler, president, Esalen Institute

ALSO BY ROLF GATES

Meditations from the Mat:
Daily Reflections on the Path of Yoga
(with Katrina Kenison)

MEDITATIONS ON INTENTION AND BEING

MEDITATIONS ON INTENTION AND BEING

Daily Reflections on the Path of Yoga, Mindfulness, and Compassion

ROLF GATES

ANCHOR BOOKS · A DIVISION OF PENGUIN RANDOM HOUSE LLC · NEW YORK

⚓

AN ANCHOR BOOKS ORIGINAL, DECEMBER 2015

Copyright © 2015 by Rolf Gates
Photographs © Arica Grafton

All rights reserved. Published in the United States by Anchor Books, a division of
Penguin Random House LLC, New York, and distributed in Canada by Random
House of Canada, a division of Penguin Random House Canada Ltd., Toronto.

Anchor Books and colophon are registered trademarks of
Penguin Random House LLC.

Cataloging-in-Publication Data is available from the Library of Congress.

Anchor Books Trade Paperback ISBN: 978-1-101-87350-2
eBook ISBN: 978-1-101-87351-9

Book design by Jaclyn Whalen

www.anchorbooks.com

Printed in the United States of America
10 9 8 7 6 5 4 3 2 1

FOR JASMINE AND DYLAN

Live your questions now, and perhaps even without knowing it you will live along some distant day into your answers.

Rainer Maria Rilke

Alignment Defined

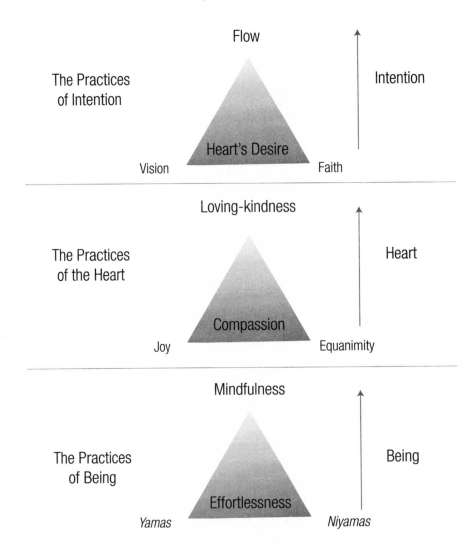

The Practices of Intention

Flow

Intention

Heart's Desire

Vision   Faith

The Practices of the Heart

Loving-kindness

Heart

Compassion

Joy   Equanimity

The Practices of Being

Mindfulness

Being

Effortlessness

Yamas   *Niyamas*

The Practices of Intention

1) Write down your heart's desires and reflect on them often.
2) Hold these intentions in your heart steadily, undisturbed by life's duality.
3) Choose faith and flow over fear and control.

The Practices of the Heart

1) Compassion: The felt experience of the desire that all beings be free from suffering.
2) Loving-kindness: The felt experience of the desire that all beings be safe, healthy, happy, and free.
3) Equanimity: The felt experience of a steadiness and composure that is undisturbed by life's ups and downs.
4) Joy: The felt experience of finding joy in others' happiness and success.

The Practices of Being

1) Effortlessness: The subtle effort it takes to be here now.
2) The *yamas*: The ethical boundaries of yoga (nonviolence, truthfulness, nonstealing, moderation, and nonhoarding).
3) The *niyamas*: The disciplines of yoga that create and sustain our freedom (purity, contentment, zeal or austerity, self-study, and devotion to a higher power).
4) Mindfulness: The art of paying attention and the practice of living with an open heart and an open mind, seeking only to know what is true here and now.

The Eight-Limb Path of Yoga

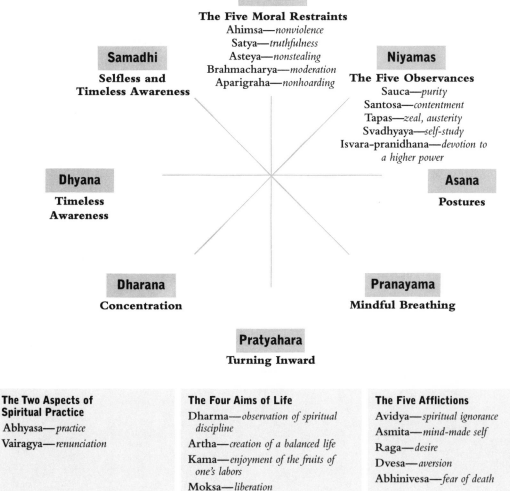

Yamas

The Five Moral Restraints
Ahimsa—*nonviolence*
Satya—*truthfulness*
Asteya—*nonstealing*
Brahmacharya—*moderation*
Aparigraha—*nonhoarding*

Samadhi

**Selfless and
Timeless Awareness**

Niyamas

The Five Observances
Sauca—*purity*
Santosa—*contentment*
Tapas—*zeal, austerity*
Svadhyaya—*self-study*
Isvara-pranidhana—*devotion to
a higher power*

Dhyana

**Timeless
Awareness**

Asana

Postures

Dharana

Concentration

Pranayama

Mindful Breathing

Pratyahara

Turning Inward

**The Two Aspects of
Spiritual Practice**

Abhyasa—*practice*
Vairagya—*renunciation*

The Four Aims of Life

Dharma—*observation of spiritual
discipline*
Artha—*creation of a balanced life*
Kama—*enjoyment of the fruits of
one's labors*
Moksa—*liberation*

The Five Afflictions

Avidya—*spiritual ignorance*
Asmita—*mind-made self*
Raga—*desire*
Dvesa—*aversion*
Abhinivesa—*fear of death*

ACKNOWLEDGMENTS

I would like to first acknowledge my wife, Mariam, for her unwavering support of me over the last twenty years, and this last year in particular. This book would never have happened without you. Next I would like to thank my agent, Carol Mann, and everyone at Anchor Books, particularly LuAnn Walther, who gave me the chance to write another book, and Tom Pold, who trudged through six months of edits. You all have my heartfelt thanks. Also, I would like to thank my many benefactors, first and foremost my mom and dad for their willingness to show up with heart and determination every day I've known them—love you guys. I would like to thank Bill W. and all his friends for a life second to none, and the Spirit Rock community for a practice second to none. I would like to thank the U.S. Army in general and the instructors at the U.S. Army Ranger School in particular for the flawless way they took me in as a clueless young person and set me on a path to a life of dignity, honor, and service. I will never forget what you gave me. Then there are the many friends who have shared their wisdom and laughter with me as I learned my way through the last ten years. My yoga friends: Nikki Myers, Johnny Gillespie, Cara Bradley, John and Chris Yax, Jacqui Bonwell, David Vendetti, Todd Norian, Patty Ivey, Toni Gilroy, Amber Favaregh, April Umek, David Sims, Grace and Mylinda Morales, Bart Daniel, Mia Oramous, Tammy Cervantes, Gaynell Collier-Magar, Heidi Sormaz, Taylor and Philippe Wells, Amber Hayes, Tracy Treu, Sean Guinan and Amy Seidewand, Theresa Murphy, Kyra Strasberg, Tommy Rosen, Matthew Sanford, David and Augusta Kantra, and Shannon and Frank Ball. Thank you to the Santa Cruz bros: Kevin DiNoto, Girish, Chad Mulder, and Hugh Burnham. A special thanks also to my wellness coach, Greg Amundson, and my photographer, Arica Grafton. I would also like to thank my children, Jasmine and Dylan. You are the greatest companions I have ever known, you inspire me to no end, and it is just the best thing ever to be your dad. And, of course, to the God of my sobriety for every breath of this life. *Namo nama*, I bow, I bow.

CONTENTS

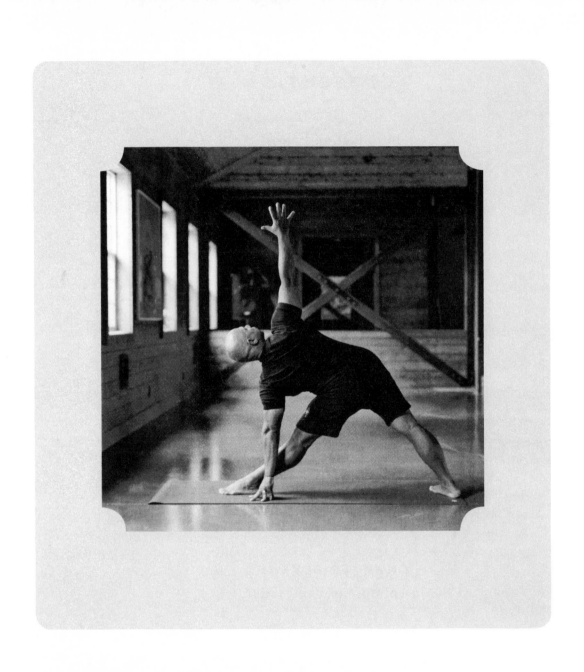

INTRODUCTION

Why This Book Now

Meditations from the Mat came to me as I was walking home after teaching a yoga class. It was a beautiful morning; the sky was mostly blue, the leaves a vibrant blend of orange, red, and brown. A student stopped me on the street to say that I should write a book. She told me that she was a writer and editor and that over the weekend it had come to her that I should turn the stories I tell in class into a book. Her name is Katrina Kenison, and I will be forever in her debt.

Talking that day on a Cambridge sidewalk, Katrina and I were in the midst of something new and beautiful, the widespread adoption of yoga poses as a means for achieving health and wellness. What Katrina appreciated was my use of stories to link the physical practice of the poses to the spiritual practice encompassed by yoga's eight-limbed path. *Meditations from the Mat* was intended to accomplish the same thing for students who would never have a chance to practice with me. As I sat down to write, I envisioned people finding something special in a yoga class at the gym or at a yoga studio and wondering how they could take that experience off their mat and into their world. It was a book about starting out and starting over, and as such it has had relevance far beyond yoga. People have written to me about how they have used *Meditations from the Mat* to help them through divorce, disease, and addiction. That I have been a part of people's lives in this way means more to me than I could possibly put into words.

In the years since I wrote *Meditations from the Mat*, I've traveled around the world, teaching and meeting with thousands of people interested in yoga. Listening to the ever-changing needs of my students and to my own evolving understanding, it has become clear to me that the initial phase in the adoption of yoga by the mainstream, in which it was primarily a physical practice, is passing, and that more and more people are looking for something deeper. My sense is that students are ready to apply the full spectrum of the practice to their daily lives—but they need help. How do we change? How do we live well and love well if it means responding with wisdom and compassion in moments when we have always reacted with fear and anger? How do we turn the purity of our heart's intention into an authentic way of being? For me, the answer to these questions is discovered when someone learns to enact and embody the teachings of Patanjali's Yoga Sutras—a series of lessons on the nature of the human condition, human potential, and how that potential can be realized that organize the essence of all spiritual practices into a basic plan for living—and the Buddha's instructions on mindfulness and compassion. *Meditations on Intention and Being* will provide readers with an ancient set of instructions for how to live and love well today. A set of instructions that takes the life we are living, the gifts we've been given, and creates happiness and freedom.

Returning readers will find this book a great companion to my earlier writing, but those unfamiliar with *Meditations from the Mat* need no prior knowledge. I will guide you through important concepts in a clear and carefully organized manner, illustrated with many examples from my own life and the lives of friends and colleagues. Whether you are an experienced yoga practitioner or you've never taken a class, whether you already meditate or you've never tried, whether you belong to a religious organization or not, you will find in these pages guidance and practices that have the ability to effect positive change in every facet of your life.

Meditations on Intention and Being is a very personal book for me, growing as it has from my own experiences and my own journey, as a practitioner of yoga and as a human being. As such, I feel it only right to share a little about my own life, so that you can understand where I am coming from and so that you can see how yoga has helped me find peace and happiness.

My Story So Far

I cannot explain why children suffer; I only know that for a number of days I walked in darkness and then one day I began to walk toward the light. There are many things I can point to that made a difference—the love of my family, the abilities passed on to me by my ancestors, the efforts of those around me to make the world a better place—but I will start with what is learned when you fall down and get back up. Because mine is a story of becoming strong in the broken places, of wrong turns leading to the right paths, and of the grace that is nowhere to be found yet nourishes and completes all things.

Learning to Learn

I spent my first two years being cared for by nuns at an orphanage in my family's hometown. Although they lived nearby, my family never visited because my skin was too dark. Later I would suffer from the same unwillingness to see or to love what was mine. At age two, I was adopted into a white community and grew up feeling like a zebra among horses. The only men I knew who looked like me were athletes on TV, so it felt inevitable that I become one too.

I played every sport but nothing really stuck until the season when I didn't make the freshman basketball team. Shocked and saddened, I let a friend talk me into trying out for wrestling instead. Walking out onto a wrestling mat to meet life honestly was the first truly courageous thing I had ever done, and it left an impression. Through wrestling, I developed a passion for discipline, process, and virtue. The army seemed to offer much of what was working for me in athletics, and after high school I decided to pursue a military career.

In the army, I learned how to learn. Before that, I was not really awake when someone was trying to teach me something, but the army used the simple device of extreme consequences to make me a passionate learner. Every day that I teach others to embrace a process and to learn through the obstacles in their path, I am merely following in the footsteps of the coaches and the military trainers who took the time to help a young person whose jumbled inner life made it hard for him to pay attention. With no more than an average grasp of what I was taught in my youth, I have been able to turn the greatest challenges of my life into a path that has led to yoga and to a life second to none.

Falling Down

I found drugs and alcohol at fourteen and loved them immediately. Despite the best efforts of my parents and my coaches, I experienced life as a stranger in a strange land. The consequences that came with my addiction felt like a small price to pay for the relief I experienced after a few beers. I spent the next twelve years exchanging whatever value I had created in my life—the relationships, the skills, the opportunities, the physical and mental health—for that relief. Mornings—waking up each day to find out what I had traded in for another few hours of not feeling—became very difficult. By the time I had an adult body, the child in me had had enough of living.

I was taken to a twelve-step meeting, where I listened to people for an hour or so. Later I prayed and my sober life began. Not drinking, prayer, and listening were my primary activities for the next few years. I got jobs and paid rent but mostly I listened, prayed, and learned how life worked one small miracle at a time. I was walking away from great suffering, and when I wasn't at meetings or at work I contended with what felt like a permanently broken heart. I have never lost the joy this pain taught me, to take in the most ordinary forms of happiness.

Getting Back Up

At the meetings I attended there was a strong emphasis on showing up for everyday life with humility, skill, and gratitude. The idea was to pour your new life into a path of service, sharing the love and beauty you found in sobriety with others as a way to keep it fresh. It made sense to me and filled me with an enthusiasm for living. I spent some time as an emergency medical technician and eventually became an addiction counselor. Getting better had become a compelling focus in my life, and I wanted to be wherever that was happening. At five years sober I got my wish and began working in residential treatment for adolescents with behavior disorders. The intensity of this work brought into stark relief the relationship between taking care of myself and taking care of others. In twelve-step meetings, I had learned that when I helped others get better, I got better. My work with adolescents revealed that I could not help anyone get better unless I got better myself. Faced with the paradoxical nature of the life I wanted for myself, a life of service, I turned to yoga.

Intention and Being

In twelve-step meetings, I had learned to live on purpose: to embrace ethical integrity and to actively cultivate insight into the truth of the way things are. Kindness and generosity were modeled as ways of life, and faith was held out as a practical alternative to fear. It was an education second to none. It was an intention second to none. The people who taught me yoga showed me how to turn the gratitude that was forming in my heart into a way of being. They embodied an understanding of life that included the experience of the breath moving through their bodies and the way the earth felt under their feet. Rooted in the stillness of the body and the rhythm of breath, I discovered the freedom that is humanity's true nature. Within the sacred spaces of yoga I found freedom from time, freedom from self, and freedom from my own ideas. I was taught to pour all the love that was rising up within me into the way I saw a leaf or felt the sunlight on my skin. The nourishment I could receive from my day-to-day experiences grew exponentially. My work with adolescents required all I had to give. Yoga taught me where to find more.

Darkness into Light

I was living the dream. I was learning to create healing spaces for children in pain, I was leaving behind the victim identity of my active addiction, and I had met the woman I would marry. The pace of growth and change in my life was picking up, but the dream had a shadow. Many of the children I was working with suffered from PTSD, and their pain revealed the extent to which I had not dealt with my own traumatic history or how it was affecting my life. Yoga became the place where I went to sort all this out. On my mat and on my cushion I found the inner space to work through the jumble of reactions that my new life inspired on a daily basis.

The traumas of my childhood had left me with an inability to feel safe or settled. Yoga has taught me how to feel both, not as a result of a circumstance but as a practiced way of being. Trauma robs us of much of the brain development that should take place in childhood, and addiction makes a bad situation worse. Yoga first helped me to address the fact that my brain often did not work well when it came to gauging reality, and over time yoga facilitated the brain growth that is associated with higher brain functioning. Yoga has made me smarter and wiser and has taught me how to feel safe and settled within the uncertainty and impermanence of life. My subjective experience of this process was of a painfully slow crawl toward being the person I aspired to be, but things actually came together fairly quickly. Within just a few years of becoming an addiction counselor, I got married and went to grad school to become a social worker. I had a plan.

Social Work

The community of healers that is social work perfectly expressed my desire to be of service. The field as I experienced it in New England in the nineties combined high intellectual rigor, compassion, and humility. If there was a downside to it all, I would have to say that it was how high the bar was set. Those people had standards. Working in anonymity, for very little pay, my colleagues performed miracles of healing, kindness, generosity, community, vision, and leadership. It was endlessly inspiring to witness what my peers were prepared to do on behalf of their fellow human beings and the feats of courage and growth their efforts inspired in the people they served. I was all in. I had found a home, and yoga was my way of keeping up with a community that was aiming to achieve the fullest expression of human potential.

In 1994, I applied to the Smith College School for Social Work and did not get in. They asked me to get more experience, so I did. In 1997, I reapplied and they accepted me. The years of work I had put in to gain this acceptance were a testament to the tenacity my twelve-step community had taught me.

Smith was everything I hoped it would be. My professors were excellent; my peers were dynamic, fun, and very bright. The only problem was that I had no real way to make money during the three years I was in school. A family friend opening a wellness center asked if I would be willing to teach yoga. I looked into it and it turned out to be the perfect part-time job while I was at school. After my first semester I received a paycheck from the wellness center and proudly showed it to my wife. I had found a way to mitigate the financial strain going to school in my thirties had placed on our lives.

When the Teacher Is Ready

The days before teaching my first class, I was very nervous. The morning afterward I was elated. Walking around my apartment, I felt as if my feet were floating several inches off the ground, and I decided that teaching five days a week would get me used to the highs and lows of the experience of teaching. I taught in a boardroom, a karate studio, a wellness center, and someone's living room. By day I worked as a mild-mannered social work intern in chinos and a button-down; by night I roamed the streets of Boston as a yoga teacher in tights, delivering wellness to those in need. Before long I began to see teaching yoga as a form of social work in itself. In particular, I loved how yoga combined the sacred with the physical for people who had often lost touch with both.

For a while I was of two minds. The space yoga provided felt optimal for the kind of work I wanted to do, but the ethical and philosophical commitments of the nonprofit world inspired me as well. It felt like my heart was in social work but my true abilities lay in teaching yoga. I eventually committed to bringing what I had learned in social work into my yoga teaching. I saw the for-profit yoga studio as a place where a community could form and become better together. With a bittersweet mixture of sadness and excitement, I left school and for the next ten years gave myself to that vision.

Happy Destiny

It's hard to describe what teaching yoga has meant to me. I have squandered many opportunities through youth and addiction, but when yoga teaching showed up, I gave it my all. There are a number of years that can be captured by the following scene: It's Sunday morning and there are more than one hundred people in the room. Everyone has worked hard and broken through to that sweet place where they are glowing from the inside out. There is laughter and joy in the room and I am the happy warrior smiling as I let go into the possibility we have created. It feels like it will last forever.

Knowing Change

My daughter, Jasmine, was born on a spring evening, and we brought my son, Dylan, home on a spring morning. My wife and I painted rooms. We bought strollers and sippy cups. We joined the ranks of new parents at playgrounds and tumbling classes. We discovered just how long the two hours between six and eight in the morning really are and how short "nap time" is—if it ever happens at all. Working harder than we had ever thought was possible, we experienced the transcendent miracle of forming a new family and found within ourselves the people we were born to be. As I write these words, Jasmine is sitting next to me doing her math homework, and Dylan has come home from wrestling and is working on a science project. It is the most beautiful thing I have ever known. It is a joy and purpose like none other.

Sitting Still

When my children were born it was clear that I was in a new world and new skills would be required. To be part of a family is to know the effect our behavior has on others in the most intimate fashion. The last time I was angry with Jasmine I watched her lips struggle with the words she felt she could not say. In a family, the pain we cause others is two feet away. To love well in this new world I have had to learn things my parents could not teach me. They taught me a lot of what I now use to create the home my wife and I provide for our children, but they could not teach me how to reflect on the mind rather than react from it. They could not teach me how to see the difference between a person and a behavior. They could not teach me how to forgive or how to experience the simple bliss of being. They could not teach me the self-awareness and compassion that come when we learn to sit still. For this I needed to practice meditation the way I practiced sobriety. With a lot of help I have been able to do just that.

Passing It On

The year after my son, Dylan, was born, I stopped running yoga studios and started training yoga teachers. A lot of what I am teaching now is what I learned by showing up for the love and accountability that is my new family.

Meditation has been the through line for all of it. Meeting the demands of my new family and my new work life has been possible because of what I learn by sitting still. Doing nothing and being nothing is how I am learning to do and be with love. This book is my way of saying thank you to my teachers and to my students by passing on what they taught me.

The Book's Design

This book is laid out in seven chapters. As a whole they represent a highly practical and relevant fusion of the teachings of the Buddha and Patanjali, maintaining the efficacy of their teachings while not becoming an academic tome.

I begin with effortlessness, which addresses the Buddhist concept of right effort and the yogic concept of "the subtle effort of effortlessness," as well as my own practical experience with nonattached involvement. This chapter is meant to help you avoid turning meditation into yet another competitive process and to teach you the means for using it as an avenue for self-actualization.

I then move to discussions of nonviolence and the spirit of practice. These chapters synthesize the moral precepts of Buddhism and the moral restraints of yoga, and include the Buddhist concept of right aspiration and the *niyamas*, or moral observances, of yoga. While teaching the role of ethics and attitude within these practices, I also make the case that ethics and attitude offer the individual both personal freedom and the ability to live with purpose.

The next chapter concerns the cultivation of mindfulness, which to many is the heart of the matter when it comes to meditation. Both Patanjali and the Buddha taught that we are not free until we can observe ourselves, and our lives, without the filters of our conditioning. This clear seeing is the practice of mindfulness. In this chapter, I present the substance of those teachings and their practical applications.

The following chapters are the foundation upon which the student rests as she learns to train her mind to see things as they are. I address the practices of loving-kindness as well as compassion, joy, and equanimity, which are known as the *brahmaviharas*, "the four immeasurables." Although these practices are more commonly associated with Buddhism, they also represent a major portion of the first chapter of Patanjali's Yoga Sutras. Once the student is able to see things as they are, the question becomes how to skillfully respond to life's pain and seeming imperfections. These chapters teach the *brahmaviharas* as an authentic and practical way forward for the world we find ourselves in today.

The final chapter is drawn from my own lifetime of practice. In recent years I have seen the "doing" aspect of my practice and the "stillness" aspect of my practice merge at the level of intention and being. Intention teaches the transformative power of orientation toward a positive vision for oneself and one's world. It speaks to the visionary, creative aspects of the human heart, the need to give voice with your life to the great heart within you. Being speaks to our capacity to experience the bliss of being. This chapter teaches that yoga is the practice of embodying the intentions we hold for ourselves and for our world.

Each chapter guides our attention toward a specific way of being that supports the larger intention to live and love well. For those of you who like for things to add up, read these chapters in order. You can also choose to open the book and read whatever the day brings. In either case, it is my experience that you will get the support you need to practice the ways of being that express your heart's intention.

A note on daily reflections: Taken as a whole, these essays comprise a comprehensive study of the practices of yoga, mindfulness, and compassion. Each individual essay is meant to offer you, the reader, a specific look into these practices. They are also meant to get you thinking and reflecting on your own truth concerning the issues discussed. The ultimate aim of a daily reflection is not to tell you what is true, but to encourage you to discover your own truth.

Namaste,
Rolf
January 21, 2015
Santa Cruz, California

MEDITATIONS
ON INTENTION
AND BEING

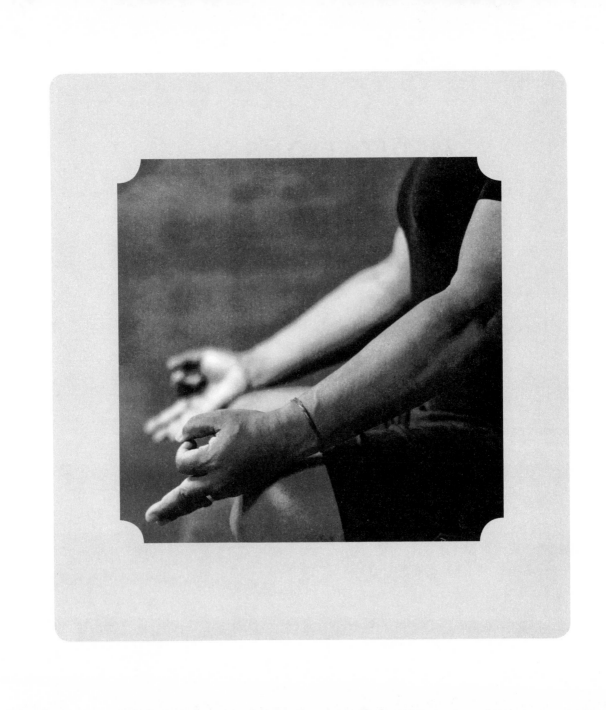

CHAPTER ONE

EFFORTLESSNESS

The pose is what you are doing.
Yoga is how you are being in the pose.

Rolf Gates

I have chosen to begin with a chapter on effort. The remainder of the book will be about things that we do and choices that we make, and I feel that it's important, before embarking on that journey, to explain that *how* we perform an action is as important as the action itself.

Sometimes, even when we apply ourselves to all the right things for all the right reasons and get good results, we continue to experience the same inner suffering that drove us to seek help in the first place. It feels as though we will never be free of a nagging inner tension, a belief that as much as we want things to be okay, they never will be. This can be a permanent state of affairs but it does not have to be. With the right support we can discover something simple and easy to remember that will alter how we approach the process of change. We come to see that how we are being is more important than what we are doing.

Doing a yoga pose while attached to a specific result is not the practice of yoga, it is the practice of attachment. Attachment focuses on the results and pulls our attention away from the process and opportunities for positive outcomes that present themselves as a moment unfolds. Starting a career, ending a marriage, or raising a family in a state of attachment to the outcome, likewise, is the practice of attachment and will yield the results of attachment. We can't free ourselves from a way of being without consciously letting go of that way of being. We must let go of what the Buddhists call our "contracted states" if we wish to experience what exists beyond them.

When I first started out as a yoga teacher, I tried to teach people to be

CHAPTER ONE

in a pose without the effort of control or attachment. These two forms of effort felt to me as if they were at the heart of most contracted states. In my own practice, when I could identify the energies of attachment and control within me and let them go, I could access inner stillness, deepen my awareness of the present moment, and arrive at an overall steadier place on my mat and on my cushion. Control and attachment were obscuring my connection to the present moment, and when I was able to let them go things improved rapidly. I wanted my students to experience this. But it is my belief that telling someone *not* to do something is not as helpful as telling someone *what* to do. So I maintained the same intention but kept refining my language. Eventually, I began to teach students to hold a pose with the intention of effortlessness.

I had been teaching yoga as the embodiment of intention for some time. I would, for example, teach students to come into the intentions of awareness and ease in their bodies, and to rest in the felt experience of those intentions. How are these intentions being expressed? Is the energy of control there? Is the energy of attachment there? I began to ask, "Can you allow the expression of those intentions to be effortless?" Spiritual practice can be understood as cultivating the habit of meeting low-energy patterns, like ill will or craving, with high-energy intentions, like kindness and generosity. This process finds its true potential when we discover the ability to hold a high-energy intention effortlessly.

Yoga finds its relevance when it can impact the way we are moving through life. My personal intention for my relationships is that I embody wisdom and compassion as I relate to my students, joy and equanimity as I drive my children to school, steadiness and ease as I sit in meditation, and loving-kindness and appreciation as I have lunch with my wife.

In my experience, I can seek to embody love while also being attached to the *results* of my actions and still trying to control others. I can create inner turmoil with the very practices that are designed to relieve it. To express an intention effortlessly empties the intention of anything extra. I can be love without attachment, awareness without control. This chapter explores the felt experience of effortlessness.

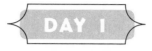

Getting Set

The air that travels across the Pacific Ocean before it reaches land has a special aliveness and sweetness to it. Breathing it feels like drinking the purest water. Waking in the early morning, I find a stillness that can be felt the way Pacific Ocean air can be breathed. Most days this stillness is the first thing I bring my conscious attention to. In the quiet darkness, I listen to it the way you listen to a breeze moving through fall leaves, breathing it in with my whole body. Taking my seat for meditation is a deliberate process. Steady in my connection to the earth (sits bones even), with a strong center (core), rooted in spirit (aware and engaged through the back of my torso), I offer my heart (shoulder integration) and align my will and my wisdom to the divine (ears over shoulders). The physical effort of coming into alignment is then transferred to the inner body, which brightens as the outer body softens. The balancing of my inner body and my outer body is arrived at effortlessly. The stillness of the seat I've taken vanishes into the stillness of the morning.

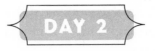

DAY 2

Knowing That I Am Sitting When I Am Sitting

Once I have taken my seat, I begin the process of letting go. The momentum that got me to my seat is no longer required in the way that walking is no longer required once you have arrived at your destination. Taking my seat is a shift from thinking to feeling. The rest of my meditation practice is a continuation of that process. The first thing I feel into is my body and the fact that I can be consciously aware of it without commentary. I spend time in the mystery of knowing that I am sitting when I am sitting. My body, and my awareness of it, brings me into direct contact with the ordinary nature of the miraculous. I am living, embodied awareness, within and expressing an eternal moment the way a wave is within and expresses the ocean. At the heart of this dynamic experience is an effortless stillness that feels like home to me.

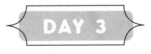

DAY 3

Just Passing Through

Connecting to stillness is like connecting to silence. We come to see that stillness and silence form the backdrop of our lives and that everything else is just passing through. Sounds come and go, sensations come and go, thoughts, emotions, all of them traveling through stillness and silence like fish moving through an eternal ocean or weather traveling across an eternal sky. As I begin my meditation, my body carries with it the experience of stillness and my mind becomes silent. I become the sky that holds the weather. Resting in the felt experience of my body, I am able to give my full attention to the weather of my life, to care for what is coming and going with wisdom and compassion, to love what is just passing through.

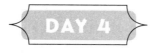

DAY 4

Life's Heartbeat

Sound travels through silence in patterns we call rhythm. Sensation travels through awareness in rhythms. Movements arise and pass rhythmically. A funny joke, a well-taught yoga class, the sound of anger, the pitch of joy, the rocking of a baby to sleep—all of it is rhythm. It is said that everything in the physical universe is information vibrating at different rhythms; the study of life amounts to the study of rhythm. Time spent in silence and stillness reveals this to be true. There is the eternal moment and there are the rhythms it holds like the sky holding weather. The first rhythm I was taught to feel into, or experience, was the rhythm of the breath. As I did so I discovered life's heartbeat. Within the rhythm of my breathing is the rhythm of all the breaths and all the heartbeats. Within the rhythm of my breathing lies the secret that I am every being and every being is me.

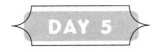

The First Breath

A friend of mine told me about a teacher who said to him, "I know the last thing you will do." My friend was taken aback, but nonetheless he asked the teacher, "Okay, what will be the last thing I do?" The teacher replied, "You will exhale." I have heard my friend tell this story a few times, and it always gets a laugh and gets people thinking. Our thoughts turn to our last breath and then, I believe, most of us reflect on our first breath. What was it like, to awaken into this world on an inhale? After a period of meditation on the body I begin to include the rhythm of the breath. Having rested in the felt experience of sitting, I begin to rest in the felt experience of sitting and breathing. As my attention moves into the breath there is always a moment of awakening to the act of breathing as I take my first full inhale.

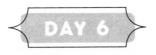

Sitting and Breathing

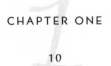

Yoga practice is intensely practical and wastes nothing. To learn about life you study movement and stillness. Walking becomes a practice, standing becomes a practice, lying down and doing nothing becomes a practice, sitting and breathing becomes a practice. In the peace of the early morning, as I let go of the need to do anything or be anywhere else, I find myself sit-

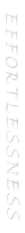

ting and breathing in the midst of a world waking up. Birdsong moving in and out of silence, cool morning air drifting on the subtlest of currents, the smell of earth and leaves wet from ocean fog, eternal silence, stillness, and space. I have a friend whose love of ocean diving began when she realized the tiny crab she was observing at the bottom of the Caribbean Sea shared a world that stretched around the entire planet. Sitting and breathing, we begin to understand the vastness of the moment in which we exist.

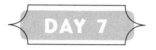

Resting

I held my son, Dylan, for the first forty-five minutes or so of his life. I watched as his eyes opened and he saw light for the first time. He looked at me and he smiled. The nurses said it could not be but it was. Once we brought Dylan home I held him in many different ways. I had a sling he could live in like a cave, a snuggly he rested in on my chest, one-armed and two-armed carries, a backpack; however I carried him we were always so close we could feel each other's heartbeats. To this day when Dylan is upset he lies on my chest so that his heart is on my heart and he just lets go. Sitting and breathing is like that for me: resting my heart in life's heart and learning to let go.

CHAPTER ONE

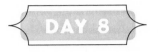

DAY 8

Becoming Available

It is said that the mind screams and the heart whispers. Over time we have lost touch with the wisdom of the heart in our efforts to manage the demands of our screaming minds. Instead of learning to listen we have learned to numb and to filter. The sensations that get through our filters and our numbness become supersized. Fear becomes violence, desire becomes gluttony, service to one's community becomes workaholism. More is never enough. Arising out of this state of imbalance is its opposite, a study of the subtle whose end point is the heart's whisper. This study is called yoga, and we make a beginning when we become available to what is happening right now. While sitting we become available to the felt experience of sitting. While breathing we become available to the felt experience of breathing. Sitting and breathing as the world wakes up, we become available to the world waking up.

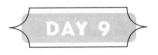

DAY 9

Plans

I tend to make a plan and then get attached to it. Anything that is not according to plan is not welcome. My time as a military officer did not lessen this propensity, nor have my years spent running the show in various capacities as a "senior" teacher. I always have a plan and so I know how things are supposed to go—according to plan, obviously. Despite a lifetime of negative consequences brought about by living this way, I did not reconsider it until my first child was born. At that point the frustrations to my plans reached an unprecedented level. Nothing about a day with a baby goes according to any plan you have ever made. My plans were a straight line and life was revealing itself to be a nonlinear series of moments. My family did not live within my lines; my wife and daughter lived in the open space of the moment. What I needed was a way to become available to a life that was a living moment rather than a plan. It was then that I discovered sitting and breathing effortlessly.

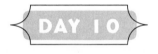

DAY 10

Learning to Swim

On my first meditation retreat I was surprised by how little instruction I received. There was a talk each night and some lecturing each morning, but for about twenty-three out of every twenty-four hours I was on my own. There was plenty of structure and accountability—we did walking and sitting meditation in forty-five-minute periods all day—but there just was not a lot of handholding and I felt some handholding was in order. Left to my own devices I began to create a routine for myself within the routine of the retreat: when I would have tea, when I would walk outside, when I would make time for some yoga poses. I found a place to take in the sunset over a snow-covered field. I learned to create a good day out of a number of good moments, my plans to give the organizers some "feedback" at the end of the

CHAPTER ONE

retreat forgotten as I sat astonished by the aching beauty of a forest quietly allowing the passage of a winter's day. By trusting me my teachers were teaching me to trust myself and to trust life.

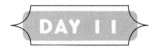

Return Is the Movement

It was not necessary for my meditation teachers to fill my days with intellectual content. In fact, that would have been the opposite of what I needed. What they were providing me with was the opportunity to see and feel something that had always been there but that I had lost touch with in the growing busyness and confusion of the echo chamber of my mind. The forest did not stage a special one-time-only winter day because I had paid to be on that retreat; the world had been effortlessly manifesting its stillness and rhythms every second of my existence. There was just a little work I had to do to be present for it. The gift of yoga is not something new; it is something being returned to us.

CHAPTER ONE

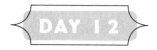

Intimacy

I do an exercise in my trainings in which I have the students enumerate the various aspects of living we negate by becoming numb to the world around us and distracted by things we do not like. The students are great at naming joy, love, adventure, understanding, and the like, but almost never mention intimacy or empathy. Yoga helps heal the fact that we live apart from ourselves, and so from our purpose and from one another. The healing of yoga usually begins on the mat and continues on the meditation cushion. We are told to balance this action with that action in the body. We are told to notice this, then notice that. We do so the way we have been trained since grade school, following instructions as we have followed instructions all our lives. Some of us are straight-A students, some of us are rebels, some of us are just not all that into it, but all of us gradually awaken to a profound understanding. Intimacy with the felt experience of the body and the breath brings peace to the mind, something we have yearned for but have despaired of ever finding. As the mind comes to rest, the heart speaks.

CHAPTER ONE

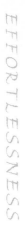

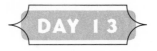

The Moment

Sitting and breathing brings us into the miraculous experience of our own embodied present moment. Over time and with practice we find that intimacy with the body and the breath exceeds the most sublime experiences of art or music. In fact, we come to the understanding that all art, all mastery, all acts of transcendence flow from and are expressions of our own inner space: the body, the breath, the mind, and the heart. As we take in the depth of our inner space we are brought into intimate contact with the larger space, the moment. There is an understanding that changes us gradually and forever. The space within us and the space around us are the same. We are the wave and the ocean—and everything else is too.

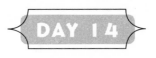

Remembering

As I sit quietly doing nothing in the cool stillness of an early morning, I remember that I am the wave and the ocean and that everything else is too. In this place fear, in any of its guises, vanishes like a shadow as the sun rises. It's not that the shadow is right or wrong, just that it has no expression in the light. In its place is a groundswell of love, understanding, and peace that is at once a call to be still and a call to action. Each breath is a wave ridden by a soul that knows itself. All that is concealed within this moment calls to me to find anew what has always been and, in this finding, to create something that has never been before. Then my mind wanders and I meet it with acceptance and compassion, returning to the body and the breath, to the cool of a world waking up and the process of remembering what I already know.

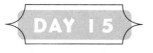

DAY 15

Forgetting

A teacher reminds the student until she remembers. Yoga serves this purpose, and yoga teachers use yoga to remind their students of what they already know. But what did we know and when did we forget it? For years, I have taught that, according to the Yoga Sutras, *avidya* (a Sanskrit term for "delusion" or "ignorance") is the root cause of human suffering. *Avidya* can be defined as a "misunderstanding concerning the way things are." This teaching has become a question I find myself living into: What is this fundamental misunderstanding, and how did we arrive at it? Nature seems to offer the most help in processing the challenge of human suffering. The natural world exists untroubled by the way things are, yet humans seem incapable of doing the same. We fret and fuss over anything and everything. We have forgotten how to be at peace with life on life's terms, a capacity my dog, Chelsea, embodies effortlessly. The ability to rest undisturbed and at ease in the timeless moment is what we have forgotten, and what yoga helps us learn to remember. When we make peace with the world as it is, it will be a peace chosen consciously, and ours will be the sweet peace of one who has known what it is to have lived without it.

DAY 16

Knowing the Body

The world I grew up in was a violent place. My country was at war, which meant very young men were being drafted and sent to their deaths. There was racial violence, domestic violence, violence as entertainment, violence as sport. The message could not have been more clear: vulnerability was a liability, and one's greatest vulnerability was one's body, with its infinity of sensations, fears, and desires. To have a body was to have problems without end. Early on I discovered all of the positive attention I could attract with my body, not to mention the array of pleasures it could bring me. My body was at once the source of some of life's greatest adventures and life's most profound pains. This was an overwhelming existential dilemma to be living into as a young person whose brain was still forming and whose culture had been warped by millennia of trauma. My first years in yoga were spent enjoying the relief it brought to the pain I had inflicted on my body. Later I would discover the relief it could bring to me mentally and emotionally as it healed my relationship not only to my body but to everything else as well.

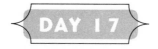
DAY 17

In the Body

Initially I approached yoga as I had football or wrestling, as a sport to master. I thought of myself as an athlete and felt confident that I could "succeed" when it came to yoga as I had on the field. I thrashed around on my mat, making things happen with as much style and dash as I could muster. The only insight I experienced came after I practiced: the walk to the car, the nap on the couch, the way I sat in a chair—things were changing in ways I could not put my finger on but I knew were related to my time on my mat. I did not succeed as a yoga "athlete," but I did injure myself often. My response to my injuries was to get upset and try to work through them. It was only when I became a teacher and saw the battles my students were having with their bodies in a pose that I began to see poses in another light. Maybe they weren't an athletic way to achieve health; maybe they were an invitation to be in our bodies in an entirely new way, completely outside of the competitive win-lose dualistic narrative we live in. Watching the violence my students were doing to their bodies made me want to stop doing violence to my own body and to be able to teach others to do the same. I began to see yoga asana, or poses, as a way to end the habit of violence, starting with the violence we do to our bodies.

CHAPTER ONE

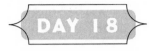

DAY 18

The First Step

We are not trying to fix something that is broken;
rather we are seeking to feel into something that is sacred.

Rolf Gates

The first step in ending the violence we do to our bodies is to move away from the belief that something is wrong with them. How would we even know if there were? It's not like we spend that much time listening to them. The bulk of our time is spent telling our bodies how they are supposed to perform and look. The shift we are trying to achieve on our mats and on our cushions is unprecedented. It is a leap of faith out of a fear-based belief system where the body is a means to an end, into a system of belief and behavior based on love and trust. Sweating away trying to fix something that is forever broken, we cannot imagine how we are ever going to feel into something that is sacred for more than a breath or two before our old fears creep back in. We do not need to know how to overcome our fear before we start trying to overcome it. We just have to take the first step, to relax, breathe, and feel.

CHAPTER ONE

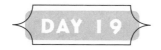

The Felt Experience

If someone asks you what yoga is, you can tell them it is a way for human beings to remember how to feel if something is true. This sounds remedial, and maybe on a cosmic scale it is, but for a species that goes to war with itself it seems like a great first step toward happiness. It's not that we weren't feeling anything before we embraced yoga, it's just that our learned mode of being is to react as opposed to reflect. With a couple of decades of yoga under my belt I recently discovered that a feeling I sometimes have is thirst and not hunger. It appears that I have been reacting to the feeling of thirst as if it were the feeling of hunger. Reflecting on this feeling instead of reacting to it has allowed me to find thirst hiding under what I thought was hunger in the same way that sadness or fear can be hiding under what we thought was impatience or anger. The process of sitting and breathing has allowed me to develop my ability to be with a feeling and to let it reveal itself to me in its own time. If someone asks me what I want or do not want, I am learning how to find the answer, and it begins with the subtle effortless action of moving from thinking to feeling.

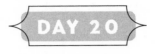

Doing and Being

Yoga offers us a set of actions to take until we are ready to try nonaction. As a species we have sought safety within an infinite number of actions, ranging from storing food for the winter to investing most of our wealth in "defense" budgets. The sum total of our actions can create a temporary form of safety, but it rarely, if ever, provides the mental and emotional experience of safety. The inner life of humanity is haunted by the implacable fact that the things we create and love are impermanent, and that the futures we are living into are uncertain. Yoga outlines a set of actions that can significantly reduce the amount of suffering we have to put up with. Living from a place of kindness and faith is highly recommended. Eventually, though, we have to take all the insights we have derived from our skillful actions and apply them to just sitting and breathing. We discover that we must practice *being* without fear if we are ever going to succeed at *living* without it.

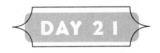

Effort and Ease

The communication that we initiate in yoga between effort and ease begins on our mats and deepens on our meditation cushions. This conversation starts with the premise that we must fix something that is broken with unwavering effort and slowly explores what happens if we let up a little. What happens if we trust life just this once? What happens if we have faith? On the mat it begins with a whole lot of effort, the same effort we have been putting forth getting to work, paying the bills, controlling this outcome, avoiding that outcome. If your teacher is skillful, the class will be just challenging enough that you can't muscle through it. The old patterns of efforting will turn out to be unsustainable. Sweating through a difficult asana session, we decide to take our teacher up on the "relax, breathe, and feel" plan. A mature asana practitioner has discovered that she can do less and accomplish more. Around that time she begins to think about meditation.

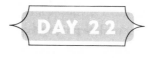

Sitting Quietly Doing Nothing

There is a moment in life when the fan of sweaty poses begins to consider meditation. It is usually after a life challenge that was endured with the help she has received from yoga. As she reflects on what got her through the divorce, the illness, or the difficult life transition, she discovers that she has arrived at an understanding that has changed her life forever. It was not what she did that got her through the difficult time; in fact, often what she did turned out to be one of the many mistakes we make during a difficult learning process. The decisive factor in her ability to grow through a moment was not what she did but why she did it. It was the intention with which she met the moment and how she embodied that intention that taught her about herself and how there was so much more to her than she knew. She has begun to see that the difficult experience did not happen *to* her but *for* her. Her yoga poses have become not so much something to do as a way to be. She has begun to understand that we are practicing ways of being all the time, sometimes walking, sometimes talking, sometimes listening, sometimes under stress, sometimes sitting quietly doing nothing.

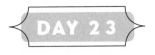

Mountain Pose

A friend once described to me her experience of studying in India with a renowned yoga teacher. She said her practice began with her standing in mountain pose day after day while the teacher gave her instruction. For a while I did not understand the teacher's decision to teach in this way. To the outward observer mountain pose is not a pose at all; the student is just standing upright, still and apparently purposeless. What I came to see is that mountain pose holds the potential of all poses within it, just as stillness holds the potential for all movement. My friend's teacher spent this time on mountain pose because if she could not achieve balanced action while standing still, she would never be able to achieve it in any other pose, and because what she learned in mountain pose she could apply to all the other poses.

I now teach students to "find their mountain" within a new or difficult pose—to find the same comfort and stability in the new pose as they experienced in the simplest one. The alignment they are seeking in their "mountain" is a harmonizing of a series of complementary opposite actions. Mountain pose—the ultimate in calm, abiding steadiness—is actually a dynamic tension arrived at effortlessly. With practice this effortless balancing of opposites can be found in any pose. The therapeutic value of this type of asana practice has to be experienced to be believed, and the physical aspect of mountain pose is only the beginning. How a student stands in mountain is how she stands in life.

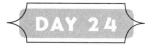

Mountain Heart

Over the years I have refined my understanding of mountain pose and of how to bring it into the way a student stands, walks, sits, and lies down. I teach the physical aspect of mountain pose whether the student is standing or sitting, then shift to the inner aspect by drawing the student's attention to what happens when we become upright in our pose or in life; as the spine lengthens, the heart opens. As we find our mountain pose we find our mountain heart. Standing calm and strong, we discover a mature capacity for openheartedness. The experience of this openheartedness, this mountain heart, is at once grounding, focusing, inspiring, and softening; it literally arrests the movement of the mind. Mountain heart delivers the felt experience of wholeheartedness, while rekindling our desire to live, love, and learn from the heart. The student standing or sitting in her mountain finds a heart that can lead her where she wants to go in life, and she learns that it will take all of her mountain pose to express her mountain heart.

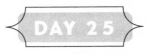

Mountain Mind

Mountain heart is spacious enough to hold the whole world and full enough to pour love into everything we do and everyone we meet, without ever running dry. It is a compass leading us to where we want to go, and it is an exquisite forest meadow to rest in all the days of our life. And before we can access mountain heart, we must first embrace mountain mind. The physical actions balanced in mountain pose require us to bring attention to many of the aspects of how we are standing or sitting that we have been taking for granted. Not only must we learn to engage muscles we have not been using, we must also relearn to use muscles we have been using incorrectly. It is an exacting process. The mind tends to become agitated as it tries to perfect this new skill. Part of the problem we encounter in finding our mountain is that the mind wants things one way or the other. Mountain pose is both and it is neither. Mountain pose is paradoxical. For example, we are filling the back of the body *and* opening the heart. These actions compete with each other, and the pose happens when we place these competing actions in harmony with each other. For the body to find harmony, the mind must learn to be present without commentary. The mind must return to its original nature, the calm spacious awareness that is mountain mind.

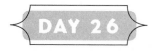

DAY 26

Mountain Moment

With the mind resting in effortless awareness, the body can arrive at effortless balance. With the body in effortless balance, the heart opens effortlessly. This is mountain moment. I tend to use mountain moment in my class the way a comedian uses a punch line. I know where I am going but I am willing to take my time and use all my resources so that mountain moment lands. Yoga students tend to show up to class having forgotten that the present moment exists and that everything they are looking for is contained within it. Their lives have become a search for something they can never find because they are looking in the wrong place and it has made them a little jaded. There is a look I often get from students that says, "Look, man in shorts, I climbed Mount Kilimanjaro on spring break while I was at Harvard, I drive my kids to the right school in the right car, and I still look hot in these Lululemons. I don't think I need you to tell me how to live my life!" And so I take my time: after thirty or forty minutes of sweaty poses I ask her to stand in her mountain. It's as if the sweat has washed away much of what has been obstructing her view. Vibrantly alive, the student stands in her mountain and feels the truth of her connection to this body, this breath, this moment, and she does it with a group of fellow human beings having much the same experience. What she is seeking and whom she wishes to share it with has been with her all along; she just had to find her mountain.

CHAPTER ONE

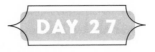

Mountain Madness

Mountain moment is so impactful that most people don't want more for a while. They are happy to "go to yoga" and find a moment or two of peace and maybe some insight. Eventually they reach a tipping point and awaken to the fact that they would prefer to extend mountain moment into mountain life. Why go to yoga if you can live yoga? At this point the search is truly on. Trainings become more trainings, poses become more poses, some folks seek more better faster, others seek more better fancy, others seek more better certain, most seek more better special, and the moment gets lost in the search. This seeking phase seems unavoidable because it is the final playing out of our faith in materialism. We have to try one more time to find some *thing* to complete our experience of *being*. We are the eternal moment seeking more. It's a paradox, mountain moment; the direct experience of wholeness produces a search for wholeness that will leave us feeling incomplete, which will, in turn, ultimately lead us back to wholeness. When the forms we sought wholeness in let us down, we begin to discover wholeness in the formless.

CHAPTER ONE

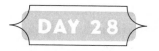

Standing Still

I read once that our species has forsaken stability for mobility. The structure of a tree expresses the preference for stability; the structure of the human body expresses the preference for mobility. We prefer to solve our problems through movement. This may explain why yoga took off in the U.S. as a form of physical exercise. My own study of problem solving began in the military, which placed a very strong focus on getting things done, on taking effective action. It was only after I stopped drinking that I began to consider the power of doing nothing. Not drinking manifested sobriety spectacularly. In fact, I was born to an entirely new way of life by not doing something. Drinking gives one result; not drinking yields an infinity of results. Movement commits us to a course of action; stillness commits us to an infinity of choices. Mountain pose is the moment in our class in which we study how we are standing in life and commit to an infinity of choices by becoming still.

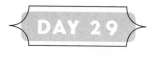

Certainty

Humanity appears to think that certainty is the natural way of things. In fact, we are willing to go to any length to control an outcome. Compulsively hopping from one action to the next, avoiding the unlimited possibilities that lie within stillness because we fear the uncertainty choice brings. We believe that it's better to reenact an old pattern whose results we know than to sit with a situation until something new arises. The preference for certainty runs contrary to the very flow of life in its infinite diversity. Life is wild with possibility and so are we. Standing in mountain pose, we remember this to be true—and the flow of life calls.

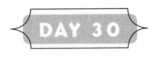

Mountain Life

Beneath our feet lies an infinity of paths. The power of mountain pose is that how we stand in it defines the path we will take and the sort of traveler we will be. The mind attempts to create a certainty about our travels, but there is none. Each time we find our mountain we choose our path forward. Each time we find our mountain we choose what kind of traveler we will be. And we cannot choose for tomorrow; we can choose only for this moment, this body, this breath.

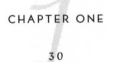

CHAPTER ONE

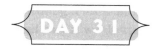

DAY 31

Standing at the Water's Edge

A year or so after I moved to Santa Cruz, California, my wife bought me a wet suit and I took the hint and learned to surf. It's even better than people say it is. At least I think so. I wake up and take the kids to school; then I pick up my buddy Kevin and we go surfing, sometimes with other friends, sometimes just the two of us. We consider a number of spots and decide on one that has a little for both of us. Once we settle on a spot we observe the ocean for a while to see what the day will bring. Watching the water is a practice that every surfer cultivates over time. The best surfers become tremendous at it. They can watch a wave and know where to place themselves on the water, which kind of board to use, and what kind of ride the wave will give them. While watching I take in the air temperature, the wind speed and direction, the swell size and direction, the effect the tide is having on the waves, and what effect the tide will have over the next couple of hours. Depending on the tide, I evaluate the level of danger or difficulty I will have getting in and out of the water (and yes, there are places I am less inclined to surf because of sharks). The real danger in this process is reducing Northern California's spectacular coastline to an equation that equals "good" or "bad" waves. Standing by the water's edge, I take in as much about what is true as I can without losing touch with the basic goodness of what I am a part of.

CHAPTER ONE

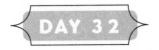

Sitting Still

One of the things you notice about experienced surfers is that they are never confused about where they need to be in the water in order to catch a wave. This lack of confusion manifests in a lack of busyness. They paddle to where they need to be, then sit still and allow the ocean being the ocean to work to their advantage. Their skill in being in the right place at the right time comes from their willingness to sit still and watch, then sit still and wait. Eventually they combine their ability to be patient and observant with the ability to act decisively, and a wave is caught. The entire process is an exquisite demonstration of doing less and accomplishing more, or to put it another way, yoga.

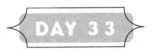

Laughing More Often

Last year I committed to meditating every day for a year. It appealed to the part of me that is still seeking "more better"; in this case, it was more better stillness. But oftentimes our more better quest gets us moving in the right direction. That was the case with my year of meditation. I feel that it is important that a yoga practitioner have some objective measure for the net gain of their practice. In my case, it is the question "Does my practice make me a better father and a better husband?" My wife is very forthcoming in this regard, so I do not have to go far looking for honest feedback. At lunch several months into my year of meditation my wife said that she'd noticed I'd started laughing more often and more deeply. She said that I found her funnier and got her humor more readily. This felt like a fantastic validation of meditation as a practice. Who doesn't want more better laughter? I believe I laugh more often because I am less troubled by the habits of my mind, and the inner space this opens up is being filled with the natural joy we all have available to us. Sitting and breathing, I take in as much about what is true as I can without losing touch with the basic goodness of what I am a part of.

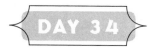

DAY 34

Doing Less and Accomplishing More

A teacher of mine described a meditation retreat he had attended in Burma during the monsoon season. His robe didn't fit properly and the one meal a day he was getting was at the bottom of a very muddy hill that he had to slosh up and down while hitching up his robe over a rapidly diminishing body. He described the meditation periods as being very long, the shortest of which was an hour and a half. At this point he paused and mentioned that he had a lot of bodily pain during the retreat. This put his own students' several well-fed dry days of meditation practice in comfortable, loose-fitting clothing into perspective. Stories like this are often interpreted incorrectly

to mean that it is only by doing more that we can accomplish more. In such an interpretation of the story the teacher was heroically taking on extreme suffering in order to achieve extreme transformation. However, the point my teacher was making with his depiction of monastic life was that he had assumed a need that he did not really have and ended up making a tremendous amount of work for himself. The choice to go on this particular retreat had been the choice for more better faster, and he had gotten more wetter painfully. The expert surfer sits still and lets the ocean being the ocean work to his advantage.

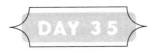

Trust

My earliest life training was in military leadership. From age eighteen to twenty-six I lived in a culture whose primary ideal was the successful execution of one's duties as a leader. At a formative age I developed a passion for getting it right when others were counting on me. The shadow side of this was the belief that I had to do everything myself and that I could only rely on life's being problematically unpredictable. Trust was just a bad idea. At age fifty I find myself with a level of responsibility that I could not have imagined as a young military officer. In the army, command responsibilities last a year or two. When you are a father, a husband, and a teacher, the term of service is indefinite, and there are definitely no weekends off. The pressures of this period of my life are more than met, however, by the efficacy of the practices I have learned in yoga. At each new bend in the road, yoga serves up the right teaching, the right teacher, the right practice to meet the new moment I find myself in, and I have learned to trust this process. I no longer have to work against life—I can sit still and let life being life work to my advantage.

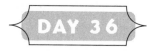

Asking the Right Questions

One of the advantages of daily meditation is that if you have some free time, several hours of sitting and walking meditation practice are enjoyable rather than a chore. Last year my schedule often had me somewhere far from home without needing to teach until six in the evening. This usually happened on Fridays, and so Fridays became my mini meditation retreat day. I would block off four hours and combine periods of sitting meditation with walking meditation and asana. One of these mini retreats took place in Vancouver, the home of the great spiritual teacher Eckhart Tolle. In his honor, I had loaded up my phone with his live talks and was bookending my silent practice with his humorous takes on waking up and letting go of the story of me. During a walking meditation period I noticed how hard at work I was. This seemed at odds with the yogic premise that we are not trying to fix something that is broken but rather we are learning to be with something that is sacred. It begged the question, what if all of this "working hard" is unnecessary? What if my mind wants to be still and spacious? I stopped walking, found an effortless mountain, and held the intention to allow my mind to rest. It did.

I spent the rest of that practice period, and all of the practice periods since then, exploring the notion that my mind is naturally still, calm, and spacious. That within this calm spaciousness lies a healthy interest in the true nature of things and that, left to its own devices, my mind will rest easy, allowing the moment to come to it. I had been asking the wrong questions, and if you ask the wrong questions, you will never get the right answers. The question isn't, how do I make my mind still? The question is, how do I stir it up? The mind is like a leaf resting on a forest floor; it takes a wind to stir it up. What causes the wind? I, me, and mine.

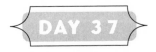

Stirred, Not Shaken

The months after my moment in Vancouver were chock-full of duties and responsibilities. I was in the midst of leading four different yearlong teacher trainings, signing a book deal, filming a ten-hour lecture series, coleading a conference on yoga and recovery from addiction, and batting cleanup at a yoga fund-raiser for Boston's Children's Hospital. At the same time, my daughter was finishing elementary school and heading off to middle school, my father-in-law was celebrating turning seventy, my wife signed her first book deal, and my dog needed to be walked regularly. Most days I get stirred up but I have never been shaken from the basic understanding that came to me that day in Vancouver. If my mind is naturally everything I want it to be and always has been, what else is too? In the midst of the everyday pressures of my life I am discovering the capacity to choose trust.

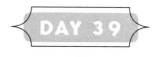

Insight

Yoga in the U.S. is all about the practice. We like to get busy and we do. We are confident in our ability to show up and get things done. We are not so confident when it comes to gaining meaningful insight from the work we put in or our ability to turn those insights into effective action on our own behalf. We come from a work-based civilization that prizes productivity and leaves big thinking to the "experts." Ours has not been to reason why, until now. I find it delightfully life affirming that despite our personal and collective preference for productivity over neuroplasticity, every human being has an innate capacity for insight into the true nature of life in general and the causes of suffering in our own lives in particular. Insight is the human capacity to see outside of our conditioned way of seeing; it is literally the ability to see what we are in the habit of not seeing. It is a natural capacity that we all share, as is the ability to put it to work in our lives.

DAY 39

First Things First

My first spiritual practice was daily attendance at twelve-step meetings and making an earnest attempt at working through the twelve steps with my sponsor. Not drinking was definitely a part of it too. I would bring myself to

CHAPTER ONE

37

meetings and spend time with my sponsor. During those "practice periods" I would hear things I had heard all my life as if for the first time. These were my first experiences of insight, and they demonstrate the working relationship between practice and insight. Once I "heard" something in this manner I could call upon this new information in order to make better choices for myself. In sobriety I found myself living into the working relationship between insight, the ability to avoid future suffering, the ongoing evolution of human consciousness, and our role in it.

One of the first insights I can remember having is into the true nature of the twelve-step slogan "First things first." It was during my first sober summer and I was living in Germany. I spent beautiful days going for runs through German farmland and summer nights talking about sobriety with other people newly liberated from the hell of active addiction. At one point I got it that if I did not drink, everything else in my life would sort itself out. Everything. I saw that there was an order to things for me. That if I wanted a great life, certain things had to happen, but one thing had to happen first. Love was great, art was great, service to my community was great, maybe even writing a book someday would be great, but none of that would happen if I drank. Sober, all things were possible. Drunk, nothing was. I saw in my heart that if I wanted anything else I had to put first things first.

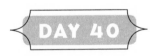

Mountain Insight

Insights are like the rainbows of our practice: we can't make them happen but they do tend to occur more often in certain places and under certain circumstances. My first real experience of rainbows was on Maui, with my wife, Mariam, during our honeymoon. Later, we spent a lot of time with rainbows in Costa Rica. Something about the balance of ocean, sun, and rain seems to appeal to rainbows. Finding your mountain is like that: it brings together all the elements that appeal to insight. You find a steadiness of body, purpose, and heart. You find an ease of being, breath, and mind. You hold stillness and rhythm like the sky holding weather and suddenly there it is: an understanding that feels like coming home for the first time.

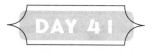

Mountain Faith

Putting insight into practice takes courage. It is, by definition, a new insight into how to live, which means that the first time we act according to a new insight we will have had zero practice with it. Not only are we new to whatever choices our insight is inviting us to make, our friends and family are new to it as well. To make matters worse, insight almost always involves love and the actions that we take to express love. And loving well can be paradoxical. We will not be taking in our addicted relative although everyone thinks we should. We will be leaving our high-paying job although no one thinks we should. We will not be listening to our fears although everyone around us thinks we should. We will be acting from love although no one thinks we should. A teacher once said, "There will never be a crowd at the leading edge." That is certainly true about the moment we take our first steps guided by insight. We will need a steadiness of heart, a clarity of mind, a firmness of purpose that we may never have had before. But that's okay because that is what our practice is for: finding our mountain.

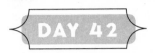

Changing Venues

Showing up to practice, whether it is on my mat or on my cushion, is a skill that requires continuous refinement. Being steady in my practice comes next. Effective practice, by definition, calls upon all our reserves of steadfast perseverance. Being available, being teachable, being honest, being kind, being generous, being adventurous, being appreciative, and being grateful are all required as well. Eventually the bell sounds and it is time to get off the cushion or roll up the mat. There is a moment of appreciation and sense of accomplishment for having done something so sweet and effective, so entirely aligned with my heart's desire for who I want to be and what kind of life I want to live. Before long I am in the flow of everyday life, on an errand with my wife, playing a game with my children, advising a teacher as she serves her community. I am living this moment, then this moment, then this moment. There was a time in my life when I could not see that my practice and everyday life presented the same kinds of challenges and required the same skills. That sense of compartmentalization or separateness has faded as my practice has deepened. Today when I get up from my practice period and show up for the next moment of my day I carry with me the understanding that my practice is not over, it has just changed venues.

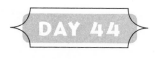

Trees

I first noticed it when I was very young. Alone in a stand of trees I could feel a vibrant presence that felt like an answer bigger than any question I knew how to ask. For a while in my twenties I spent my free time in a canoe with a friend gliding across lakes, flowing with the current of a deep-woods river, Maine's pine forests providing an energetic symphony. It felt like God and an infusion of God energy. When I wasn't on the water in an endless forest I felt lonely for it. The moments I did spend in nature were bittersweet and filled me with a longing for more. The first decade of my yoga practice felt like those canoe trips: tastes of freedom, tastes of wholeness. Meditation taught me that the trees were teaching the power of stillness and that whenever I wanted to be with the trees I simply needed to be still. Today when I think of loving-kindness I think of being for others what the trees have been for me.

Kindness

The design of our bodies expresses the preference for mobility over stability and the solutions we seek tend to involve doing something. Not only do we

CHAPTER ONE

prefer to try to act on our problems, we prefer to have as much control over the outcome of our actions as possible. This seems reasonable but it puts us in a difficult position when our greatest teachers suggest turning the other cheek, forgiving everybody for everything, and loving our neighbors as we love ourselves. Taking a kind action for the action's sake and letting go of the results. How exactly is that going to turn out?

My life was saved, sustained, and changed forever by a series of acts of kindness by people who were perfect strangers and had nothing material to gain by being kind to me. The people who helped me believed in kindness and were willing to do what they could to bring more of it into the world. The kindness they offered me had no strings attached, and I have spent every day since trying to bring kindness into the world as it was brought to me.

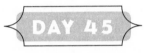

Nonattachment

Attachment can be understood as something extra and unnecessary that negates the action we are taking, like giving someone a glass of water and then drinking it for them. We can give our attention to something, give our time, give our strength, our faith, our love, our appreciation, our money, our food, even our lives; all of these are ours to give freely, but nothing has really been given until we let go. I have learned this several different times in several different ways. Teaching teachers, it became clear to me that I needed to offer them what I knew, then let them decide how they were going to use my example. Loving my wife, my children, and my friends is something that is done unconditionally or not at all, no strings attached. Sitting and breathing is just sitting and breathing, nothing else. Sitting quietly in the cool of a world waking up, I can feel when there is a little extra effort, an attempt at control, the effort of trying to add to something that is already complete. When I let go of control, when I allow my sitting to be effortless, when I become empty, the fullness of the moment is available to me.

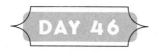

Fearless

I live on the side of the Santa Cruz Mountains and hike in them often. When it's just me and my dog, Chelsea, I will hike for five minutes or so, then stop and find my mountain. In the silence I feel the forest breathing with me. Then I walk on for a while before I stop and find my mountain again. In the silence I feel the forest breathing with me. Then I walk on for a while before I stop once more and find my mountain. In the silence I feel life breathing me.

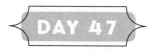

Right Effort

Before I began teaching yoga I'd been gifted with talent and opportunity. I went to good schools, received great coaching in sports, won scholarships,

CHAPTER ONE

43

was given a commission in the U.S. Army and a small fortune in military training. But despite these resources, my potential did not come to fruition due to an addiction to alcohol that claimed me early in life. By the time I began teaching yoga I had been sober for a while and had had the chance to feel the sting of the many opportunities that had passed me by. With yoga I had another chance. In yoga I was not going to be a talented person; I was going to be an all-in person. I knew that there was no telling how things were going to go, that there was no reason to believe that I would be any good at teaching, but that was okay. Yoga was not going to be about success or failure; it was going to be about giving everything I had every minute of every day. As an athlete I had competed to win something for myself; as a teacher I have done all that I can to give something back. In the years between my last drink and the first yoga class I ever taught I had seen death and chosen life, and I was going to live accordingly. Nearly twenty years later I still feel a boundless joy every time I get to do the best I can on behalf of something that I love. When people thank me, I mean it when I say that it is my honor and pleasure.

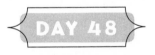

Right Intention

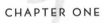

I cried at my graduation from rehab. My old life was over and the new life I was beginning was more beautiful than anything I had ever imagined. My tears were a combination of grief for the life I had lived and joy for the life I had just begun. When I got back to the infantry battalion that had sent me to rehab I still had official duties to perform. It was not so much a rude awakening as a struggle with an odd leftover life that I had to clean up before I could begin my new sober one. The scope of my duties was extremely familiar to me, but I was now at a loss when it came to my motivation. My old life had been driven by fear and anger, and both of them were now in short supply. Without fear and anger how did one get things done? And why? I spent a week or two breezing about my military post trying to find something solid to stand on. I was no longer afraid of anything, except going back to drinking, and life—which seemed kind of dreamy and wonderful after a sober night's sleep—made anger feel unwarranted. The departure of my anger and my fear had left a void in my life and something else started to fill it. I began to feel powerfully how dear my friends were to me. I began to feel how much I respected the senior officers in my battalion and to appreciate their decency and kindness. I now began to see life in the battalion as something I could contribute to for no other reason than the natural love I felt for my community. I found that I was standing on love and that it was a rock.

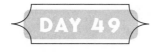

Right Intention and Right Effort

Something happens when we align our will and our heart. Our efforts become an unstoppable force for good. The joy that we take in this kind of action is not the pride of achievement, nor is it the joy of possession, for it does not belong to the realm of the separate self. The joy that is felt when our will soars on the wings of our heart is too big to belong to any one aspect of creation. It is a joy that belongs to us all. The strength we embody

CHAPTER ONE

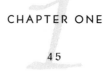

45

is the strength of us all, the kindness, the wisdom, the grace, the wit, the poetry, the vision, the courage, the beauty that we love and create—all of this belongs to us all. For a moment we are the hand of creation, the voice of creation, the heart of creation. The ancients called this "vivid true knowledge," or "direct knowledge of the soul," and it is enough for any heart. The only reward we ever need for such an experience is to be given the opportunity to serve once again as the hand of all of us.

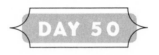

Effortless

Throughout our lives we try a number of things for any number of reasons. We try this to fit in. We try that to please our parents. We try this because we are afraid. We try that because we are angry. We try this because we are lonely. We try that because we want to be left alone. Almost everything we try costs more than it is worth because we think that it is something that it is not. Everything we pick up is empty. But some of us have found the secret to making everything full. It's called love, and an endless ocean of it lives in our hearts. The ones who know this secret say we are supposed to pour our love into all that is empty. They say that you will know that you are pouring your love into the world because it will feel effortless.

THREE WAYS TO PRACTICE EFFORTLESSNESS

1) Choose faith over fear. In practice and in everyday life, allow your choices and your actions to flow from faith.

2) Act in the service of what you are *for* rather than what you are *against*. Embrace what you are for and allow others the freedom to choose what they are for.

3) Do nothing and be nothing: this is how we learn to do and be with love. Sit quietly doing nothing and being nothing daily.

CHAPTER ONE

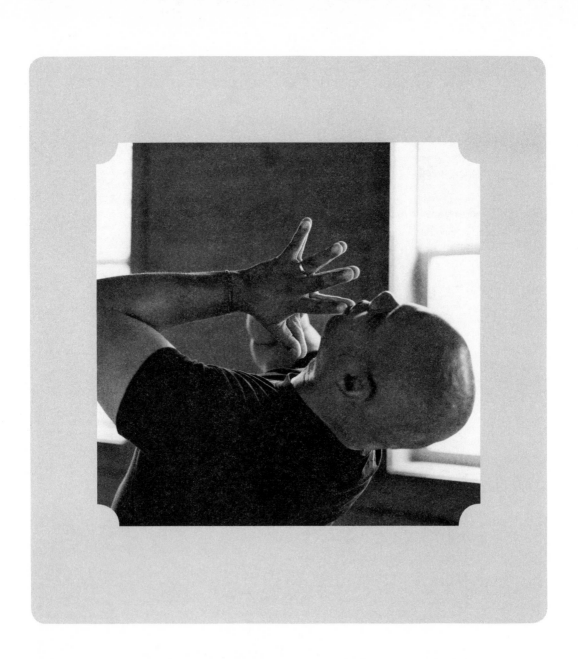

CHAPTER TWO

NONVIOLENCE

The foundation of yoga is a commitment to nonviolence. This is sometimes also called "nonharming," but for me nonviolence is the most unambiguous way to express the idea. Violence, in any form, must be abandoned, categorically, if we are going to achieve our potential, individually and collectively.

I began my own imperfect practice of nonviolence while still on active duty in the army. I was sitting in a group, during my six-week rehab, when the thought came to me that if I had not known I was an alcoholic or that there was a higher power that could relieve me of the desire to drink (as was proving to be the case), what else did I not know? It seemed clear to me that I was likely ignorant of most things that mattered. That having been said, how could I possibly know if someone's life should end? It was clear to me that, out of respect for the higher power that was keeping me sober, I should refrain from playing God by deciding who lives and who dies. That decision was way beyond my pay grade. I did not feel conflicted about my remaining time in the military; my commitments were clear and my heart was untroubled. I returned to my infantry battalion, completed my service, and treated each of my remaining days in the military as a chance to practice the principles of love and service that I was learning in sobriety with the people closest to me, my fellow servicemen and -women.

You can find fault with this kind of nonviolence, but it was a start for me, and I have not gone back. Initially the nonviolence I practiced was a form of paying respect. I'd had what, for me, was incontrovertible proof that there was a higher power that loved everything unconditionally. There was no doubt in my mind that this higher power cherished every aspect of the world: the plants, the animals, the rocks, the trees, and every person I met. It seemed that to try to act accordingly was the least I could do. The greatest happiness I have ever known has been to honor my higher power by doing right by its children.

This became my highest aspiration. The downside of this aspiration has been the inability to forgive myself when I have fallen short. It turns out that getting sober and getting my yoga on doesn't mean getting perfect. There have been very hard moments reconciling the part of me that knows love with the part of me that still lives in fear. I have learned that we are love-based beings and that the worst thing we can do to ourselves is to deny this truth through nonloving behavior. Today, nonviolence is a way to take care of myself, to respect myself, and to protect myself from the worst form of injury I can do to myself.

Over time I have come to understand the practice of nonviolence as a refinement process. Through trial and error we discover what loving well is and is not. To see our shadow we must stand in the light, and yoga provides that light in the form of the *yamas*, the five moral restraints of yoga (nonviolence, truthfulness, nonstealing, moderation, and nonhoarding). The *yamas*, together with the *niyamas*, the five observances of yoga (purity, contentment, zeal, self-study, and devotion), can be thought of as the Ten Commandments of yoga, the fundamental practices that govern how we live. By making a clear commitment to the *yamas* we create for ourselves a way to measure the merits of a choice, a pattern of behavior, an assumption. We are able to unravel the mystery of cause and effect as it pertains to what matters the most—love.

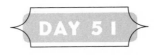

Living Without Regret

When a loved one passes, there is only one good thing you can say about it. In the pain of their passing you get to experience a form of clarity that nothing else can match. When a loved one is gone you know, really know, that all that matters is saying "I love you." Everything else is pointless in comparison. If you have had this experience, your loved one has given you a chance like none other. You get to live the rest of your life in the remembrance of what they taught you about love. This is how you love them after they are gone. This is living without regret.

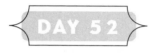

The Other Side of Love

It's as if the pain of losing a loved one, like the joys of parenting or the astonishing vibrancy of romantic love, has the power to complete our training in love. In the clarity of grief we see that there is only how much we loved them. In the clarity of grief we see that there is no other side of love. Loss has the power to touch us in such a way that we no longer see any point in working *against* when we can work *for*. We decide to leave fighting against things to those who have the time. It is only in this light that we can begin the practice of nonviolence. It is only after completing our training in love that we can begin to choose only love. Once love has truly taken hold it becomes clear that although there are many demands on us, and many competing priorities, at the end of the day there is only one thing worth living and dying for. My training was completed on a cold winter morning as I heard the ambulance coming for my sister. As I waited for the men who would come too late, I knew that our time is short; it will mean something or it won't, and love will be the judge.

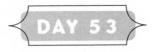

Generosity

If we are lucky, life will humble us. We will be brought low by love and gratitude and find that place within us that wants only to be kind and generous. We may not have had much practice with these feelings, but we are willing to learn. We find that whatever time we have left we are more than willing to devote to learning how to love well. There is usually something we can do: a volunteer position, a training we can take; for some of us it is a yoga class to teach. Once we have embarked on a path of service, however humble, we find that we have bound ourselves to a path of self-awareness. If we want to be truly helpful we must learn to get out of our own way. The heart awakens the desire to serve; the desire to serve awakens the desire to serve wisely.

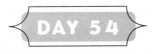

Giving and Receiving

I was taught that there are two aspects of yoga: sitting quietly and sweeping the garden. This idea captures the relationship between service to others and the everyday practices of yoga. Sitting quietly is the inner work of yoga, sweeping the garden is the outer work. Whether we begin with the inner work by going to a yoga class or the outer work by serving our community in some way, we find that one does not last long without the other. The phenomenon of burnout in the helping professions speaks to the fact that if we don't recharge our batteries, they run out. The "ten years around yoga" phenomenon, in which students spend time around yoga without actually getting that much out of it, speaks to the need for a measurable positive from practice besides a little stress reduction and toned abs and buns. By consciously linking our inner work with our outer work, we create a synergistic dynamic of giving and receiving that makes living our yoga sustainable.

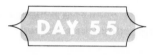

Keeping It Fun

I began linking the practices of my life with something deeply compelling early on. The first kind of training I ever undertook was getting ready for varsity football. I had seen the older kids work out with weights, and all of them talked about Nautilus equipment as offering the best range of motion. There was a Nautilus facility a mile or so from my house, and for a long, hot summer I made my way to the gym three times a week. Nautilus was in a largely windowless rectangular building in a defunct section of an industrial park. There was no AC, nor were there any attempts at décor. There was a constant clanking and grunting and the place smelled bad. AJ, the friend I began training with, dropped out within a couple of weeks and for the rest of the summer I was on my own. This was not like playing basketball with friends, swept up in the joy of the game with time flying by. If I wanted to get a workout I had to generate my own enthusiasm.

That summer I learned to create a "lifting psych" by designing new workouts and by wearing special shirts for special days. Sometimes I would jog to the gym, sometimes I would jog home; at intervals I would use a heavy bag, then a jump rope. I even invented a form of circuit training for myself about a decade or so before it became popular. This was my first real life skill, creating a meaningful practice, and possibly it's the one thing I am really good at. In the years that followed, wherever I was, whatever was going on in my life, I could always make it to the gym, my mat, my cushion. The trick seems to be to capture your own attention, to make getting to your practice something compelling, to turn the theoretical benefits of practice into a felt reality eagerly anticipated. I brought this understanding into my yoga practice, with a slight adjustment. Where once I was training to play well, today I am training to love well.

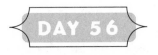

Sweeping the Garden

The Yoga Sutras state that the key to consistent practice is the awareness that we practice for ourselves and for others. In order for our practice to become truly compelling we must be able to see how it positively impacts not only ourselves but those around us as well: our family, our friends, our community. The skill that is captured in the phrase "sweeping the garden" combines making the personal growth you are experiencing in yoga of benefit to your community and finding gardens that inspire you to continue growing. It's a behavior that we see all around us. It's the father who runs a company but finds time to coach soccer because he knows the time and the effort will leave him happier in his life. The young person who has gone back to school so that she can work for social justice because her heart demands that her actions express the compassion she feels for the suffering of others. The lawyer who takes cooking classes and opens a farm-to-table restaurant because he has been touched by the importance of healthy eating. You know you are in the right garden when you would pay to be allowed to sweep it. You know that you are in the right garden when your practice feels like indispensable preparation for another day of sweeping.

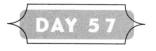

New Gardens

When my first child was born, I found myself sweeping a garden the likes of which I had never even imagined. In this garden, a good night's sleep was replaced by a good cup of coffee, vacation time was replaced by nap time (although even then my kids napped less than any other babies in the history of babies), and sitting in an unshaded spot on a bench at a theme park had to pass for "me time." Times had changed and my yoga practice had to change with them. In the past I had been able to block off hours at a time to prepare for experiences I found mentally or emotionally challenging. In this new phase of my life those types of situations came so frequently and from so many different quarters that any space I was going to find would have to be inside me. The cultivation of inner space through meditation became indispensible preparation for sweeping this new garden.

About four years into this new adventure I was on vacation with my wife and children, my parents, my sister, and her two children. We had found a good deal near Disney World and were all living in the same house. I was paying for this trip by teaching, so I found myself alternating visits to the Magic Kingdom with visits to a yoga studio in Orlando. At one point amidst the protracted mayhem I was holding my one-year-old son when he grabbed my brand-new three-hundred-dollar glasses off my face and in the blink of an eye twisted them beyond repair. My first thought was to be impressed by his hand speed and to be grateful I could afford to buy replacements. Times had changed, and so had my yoga.

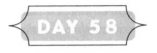

DAY 58

Sitting Quietly

The skill implied by the phrase "sitting quietly" involves matching the nature of our practices with the demands of the gardens we are sweeping. Often the practices that got us to a garden won't sustain us within it. The example that comes to mind is of the yoga teacher who has a great asana and meditation practice and is able to teach from it in a way that really helps people. This leads her to open a yoga studio. Before long her job description has changed: where once she was just a teacher, now she is also a manager. Managing takes an entirely different skill set than teaching, and often the teacher must address unexamined family-of-origin issues if she wishes to succeed as a manager. To sweep this new garden, she must find practices that help address whatever interpersonal issues she still struggles with. To effectively "sit quietly" year after year requires us to be ready to change the way we are sitting.

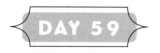

Balance

I read once that balance is actually the body harmonizing numerous micro-movements. The stillness of the body in balance is an illusion; the truth is that balancing is a dynamic process. So it is with sitting quietly and sweeping the garden. For our yoga practice to be sustained over time, and for it to stay relevant in our ever-changing lives, it must continue to evolve with us. The gardens we sweep must be worthy of our hearts, and our practices must be relevant to the demands of our gardens. The two things—our gardens and our practices—are really one thing; they are the practice of yoga.

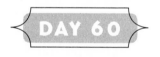

Doing No Harm

Sitting quietly and sweeping the garden set up a powerful dynamic in our lives. Whatever growth and opportunities we are seeking will invariably come to us as we live our yoga one day at a time. The life that we create in this manner will be precious to us in a way that just keeps getting better. The quality of the life we are living heightens our sensitivity, and the fallout from our own unconscious patterns becomes intensely painful. A feature of our new life is an earnest desire to do no harm. We discover the significance,

CHAPTER TWO

59

often for the first time, of the concept of healthy self-boundaries. Lao-tzu wrote, "Knowing when to stop we can avoid all danger." We find ourselves wanting to know when to stop with our bodies, when to stop with our words, when to stop with food, when to stop with money, when to stop with control, when to stop with anger, when to stop with sex, when to stop with work, when to stop with practice, when to stop with our thoughts. We find ourselves living into a paradox. Healthy self-discipline creates and maintains our freedom.

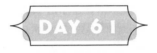

Self-Discipline

My formative experiences with boundaries came in the form of rules that were created by adults who did not seem particularly interested in my welfare. Rules held an arbitrary place in my world. The weather made sense to me, gravity made sense to me, sports made sense to me, having a pet made sense to me; rules, however, did not. They seemed to emanate from a darker dimension in which my very nature was unwelcome, and abiding by them was a form of humiliation. I grew into adolescence without any knowledge of or respect for the concept of self-discipline. I was what Bill Wilson, the founder of Alcoholics Anonymous, called a true child of chaos, and I had company. My friends and I lived within the glamour of a victim story that was too all-encompassing for us to know it for what it was. If I'm already in prison, why build walls? In sobriety and with yoga I dragged myself slowly but surely out of my story of victimhood and into the understanding that I was already free. From a place of freedom I discovered the dignity that can only be found in choosing to bind oneself to a discipline.

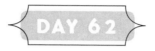

Free Will

It is not until we can extricate ourselves from the victim narratives we live by that we are able to grasp the full scope of our own free will. To let go of a victim story you have to know you are living one, and this can be tricky because they hide in plain sight. Many of us choose conventional victim narratives that are built around class, gender, race, and religion. Others are more inventive, creating reverse-discrimination narratives ("they hate us because we are free"). Some of us are victims of our parents, some of us are victims of our addictions or our health and wellness challenges. Some of us are even victims of our talents and fame. Mother Teresa was visited by Jesus Christ, then felt awful that she did not get more visits. For most of us there is a period when the glass is half-empty.

Oddly, the usual course of things is that they have to get worse before they get better. We have to go through an actual injustice before we can stop keeping score and start living free. A divorce in which a cheating spouse is vindictive and gets most of the money, business partners who sue and slander to get more than their share, a random and life-threatening health crisis, siblings who freeze us out of the family fortune—the list is as long as it has to be for us to stop waiting for things to get fair before we start living. Presented with an actual injustice, we arrive at the realization that every moment we wait for justice, a poorly defined entity at best, is a moment that we are giving our power away to a situation instead of living the life we choose.

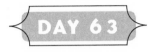

The Price of Freedom

The price of freedom is the abandonment of blame. To abandon is to walk away and not look back.

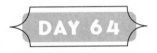

The Practice of Choice

Choice arrives in stages. It starts out with a lot of conditions. *If she does this I will have no choice but to do that. If he does not do this I will have no choice but to respond in kind. You made me so angry, I cheated on you because you were distant and unavailable. If you had my problems you would drink too.* Our ability to choose is tangled up in a lot of circumstances that are out of our control. Yoga heightens our sensitivity, and we become increasingly uncomfortable with both our willingness to avoid responsibility for our actions and the consequences this avoidance is raining down upon us and the people in our lives. We arrive at the desire to be courageous and responsible in life, to step up and stand for something. This is an important development, and often hidden in it is the belief that if we do the right thing the world will conform to our sense of fairness and justice. Then we reach the critical stage: life chooses not to conform to our ideas of fairness and justice and we discover that it does not matter; what matters is what we choose to do. Then yoga starts to transform our lives.

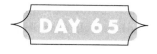

At the Beginning

At the beginning of the Buddhist meditation retreats I attend we commit to a set of ethical precepts that are several thousand years old. Despite the fact that we are about to spend a protracted period of time in silence without any practical interaction with one another, it always feels like a big deal to formally vow to play by the rules of the community we are choosing to be a part of. The retreats are arduous, featuring walking and sitting meditation in silence from before sunrise to well after sunset, and it feels like taking the vow at the beginning is critical to my success. Without the commitment to being accountable to my community I do not think I could be successful in my efforts to be accountable to myself.

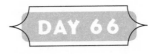

Discipline and Freedom

A teacher once told me that it is only by making a clear commitment to a spiritual principle that we are able to break free from our patterns. Once we make a clear commitment, the work we must do to unlearn an old pattern and practice a new one begins. I gave an assignment to a group of teachers to commit to one of yoga's ethical precepts for a month. They found the experience so revealing that they kept it going for the remaining four months of the training. What they found was that they had been avoiding, controlling, or numbing some aspect of their experience, and the conscious practice of an ethical discipline forced them out from under the cover of their avoidance strategies and into a more direct connection with themselves and the people in their lives. This direct, authentic connection had been what they were looking for when they came to yoga in the first place. A new discipline had provided them with a new freedom.

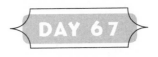

Avidya

The Yoga Sutras state that the root cause of our suffering is a fundamental misunderstanding. This intuitively made sense to me when I was first learning about yoga, but what was the misunderstanding? If it is the root cause of all human suffering it should be pretty obvious, right? What was it? Is the world really flat? Am I misunderstanding misunderstanding?

A few months before I sat down to write this book my biological mother contacted me. She had dropped me off at an orphanage when I was ten days old, and at two I was adopted and raised by the people I think of as my parents. It was clear that she had thought through her decision to contact me and that she meant well and was willing to answer my questions patiently and honestly. Nevertheless, her return precipitated a physical, emotional, and mental crisis. My lower back seized up and an old army injury to my Achilles tendon flared up simultaneously. As I worked through the pain in my body and my heart I saw that what was required of me was that I be willing to have this experience without fear. I saw that stored within me was the assumption that certain aspects of my life had to be managed, controlled, or denied and that this effort was causing my pain. For the pain to end I had to stand in it without fear. I saw that *avidya*, or our "misunderstanding concerning the way things are," is the mistaken assumption that we should be afraid of life.

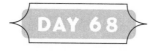

Freedom from Fear

The assumption of fear and the logic of fear must be deconstructed methodically. My moment working through the pain of my mother's return came on the heels of a quarter century of work in which I systematically brought awareness to every aspect of my life. Years of bringing attention into the body and the breath, years of watching the mind, years of practicing ethical living, years of service to others, all of it slowly eroding the assumption of fear so that when I was in a "crisis" I could understand it for what it was: something I had learned to be afraid of, something I misunderstood. I could feel the physical, emotional, and energetic presence of fear and my efforts to control it, and I had learned to question the logic of fear. I had learned to stand fearlessly and effortlessly in my mountain. Once I was willing to do this the truth of my history with my mother, which had been repressed energy, was allowed to be reintegrated. What had been a terrible pain became a simple message: do not be afraid of this or anything. The phrase that arose as I let go of my fear and the energy moved through me was "Know this now." Now is the time for us to live without fear.

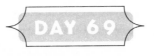

One Small Step

One might draw the conclusion from my last reflection that the path of yoga is a series of epic mountaintop battles with core pain. It is not. Most of the time it is a series of ordinary moments in which we seek only to know what is true and to take a small step in truth's direction. The design of yoga's eight limbs can be understood as a set of circumstances in which to study the contents of our life. One circumstance is the fact of breathing. What is true about the act of breathing now? One circumstance is the phenomenon of thinking. What is true about my thinking now? The practice of nonviolence does this for us as well. What is true about the way I am relating to this situation? Am I being kind, is my speech wise, am I being generous, am I acting in a way that supports the relationships in my community, am I acting from a place of abundance or scarcity? The commitment to nonviolence allows us to bring our attention into our everyday life and systematically deconstruct the logic of fear.

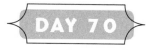

Meeting the Moment

The first of the eight limbs of practice laid out in the Yoga Sutras is called the *yamas*. These are the ethical precepts of classical yoga and serve as the energetic foundation for the rest of the limbs. The idea is that if you are lying, cheating, and stealing it doesn't really matter if you can stand on your head in a pose. You have bigger problems. If, however, you are in right relations with yourself and your world, inner peace and personal growth are reasonably attainable if you are willing to work toward them. The work of right relations itself requires us to apply yogic principles with both wisdom and compassion. The person who is working all five *yamas* in her life has aligned herself with the flow of life. Nonviolence is both the first of the five *yamas* and the overarching intention of them all. Wise speech, nonattachment, generosity, and the appropriate use of our sexual energy are all merely expressions of the desire to live from a place of nonviolence and kindness.

DAY 71

The Block

Einstein wrote that humanity lives imprisoned by a mind-made sense of separation, and that to free ourselves from this prison we must widen the circle of our wisdom and compassion to embrace all of humanity and the natural world. Yoga can be understood as a plan for such a widening. To be practiced properly, every aspect of yoga must be understood in this light. *Satya*—"truthfulness" or "honesty"—is the second of the five *yamas*. It begins with our ability to reflect honestly on our own inner life and our own felt experience.

For many of us, our first moment of *satya* is when we choose a modification in a yoga pose. The pointlessness and the discomfort of trying to get into a pose that is not appropriate for our body becomes apparent to us. We pick up the block we have held in contempt and find a more accessible and more productive version of the pose. By being honest about our experience of the pose we find that doing a little less allows us to accomplish a lot more. From the very beginning honesty is something we practice from the inside out.

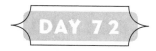

The Appearance of Things

As children we learned about the world from the outside in. The name of things really mattered. If you knew the name of something you knew what it was. It was almost as if knowing the name of something was the same as understanding it. *That's a chair, that's a dog, I'm a boy, she's a girl.* We learned to label things and then respond to our labels. As parents we tend to applaud this process, encouraging our kids to name everything around them and reinforcing the idea that labels matter. Unfortunately, our labels can be the bars of our mind-made prison. The first time this became clear to me was when I considered how it felt to be labeled a racist term, how someone calling me a name had the power to make me feel awful. Later, the grade I received on a test was so important I thought nothing of cheating to get an A. The name someone called me or the letter on my test had the power to define me.

The world of labels was also extremely confusing. Things tended not to add up. Killing is bad, so we like to kill killers. We are all God's children, except those people over there. Trying to arrive at the truth using labels turns out to be a dead end. Many of the things we were taught would make us happy don't. We find that we no longer have the ability to settle for the appearance of things. We find that we don't just want the appearance of having a life; we want the experience of it.

CHAPTER TWO

2

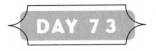

DAY 73

Moving from Thinking to Feeling

A rule of thumb in my yoga teacher trainings is that "a principle felt is a principle understood." The yoga teacher articulates a principle, then provides the student with a felt experience in which to apply the principle in order to understand it. For example, I will discuss the interaction between the physical body and the energy body, then we will do several simple exercises that demonstrate that proper alignment facilitates the flow of energy in a pose and that an energetic intention has the ability to organize the physical body in a pose. The physical practice allows the student to take a concept off the whiteboard and into her body. She begins to discover what is true for her by moving from thinking to feeling. Later, when she is presented with a choice, the feedback given to her by her physical body and energy body starts to inform her decision. Eventually she learns to trust this feedback more than the two-dimensional labels she has learned to apply to life.

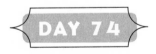

DAY 74

Getting Honest

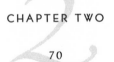

Getting honest is a process. The innate intellectual dishonesty of labeling things and then reacting to our labels hides in plain sight, and it takes a trained eye to see it for what it is. Our labels give us a sense of certainty.

This is good, that is bad, this is safe, that is not. Most of us have stayed in unhealthy relationships to avoid the pain of ending them. I believe we have a similar relationship with our labels. We treat our labels like they are people, making it hard for us to walk away from them. Leaving a label is often felt to be a betrayal of the person or the group of people who taught us the label. Your beliefs honor your mother's spiritual beliefs, but are you still a good daughter if you no longer affiliate yourself with her church? In order to skip over the pain of loss and the uncertainty of being without a label, we often just change definitions: we go from being a Christian to being a Buddhist or a yogi, never having to examine the dysfunction of the labeling process in the first place. This is why the felt experience of the body and the breath is so central to the process of getting honest. Sitting and breathing, we experience directly that there is no time, no life to divide into past and future, only now. Sitting and breathing isn't hard or soft, hot or cold, good or bad; it's all of these, and more. Life includes and transcends all labels, and yoga is a way of remembering this.

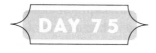

Being Honest

The importance of being honest is something we knew all about as children. Lying felt bad. Later we retreated from our physical bodies, our emotional bodies, and our energetic bodies, and the pain of being false became a distant echo in the back of our subconscious. I remember a young Harvard Business School student telling me she was sure that there was a net positive to war. I conceded that she might be right; who knows these kinds of things? And

I told her that yoga would have her spend time in combat to determine the truth of war's value. Adults tend to believe that merely thinking something is enough to make it true. Being honest means being willing to feel into the truth of something. We don't start with big stuff like the net positive of war; we begin with something simple and close by, like the quality of effort we put into standing and walking, or sitting and breathing. My teachers tell me to be right there at the beginning of each in-breath. They teach me to be honest about my connection to the in-breath and the out-breath. Later, if we have worked hard with the breath, we will begin to feel if we are right there when a loved one is talking to us. We will know if we are right there as we make a choice or take an action. We will know if we are right there as life is happening.

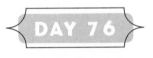

John Wayne

I grew up on John Wayne movies, and to be honest, despite his shortcomings, I have seen far worse role models. John Wayne was brave and loyal. He worked hard, but always for family, love, or country, never for money. The violence, racism, homophobia, and misogyny of his time were well represented in his movies, but they were well represented everywhere back then. The real problem with John Wayne as a role model was that he was an actor in movies, not a real person making meaningful choices in the real world. John Wayne's characters dealt in black and white; life happens in shades of gray. My early efforts at living life John Wayne–style kept rubbing up against the fact that nothing I could give myself to was as simple

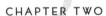

as it was in the movies. The people I dealt with weren't all good or all bad either. And, most challengingly, I was neither purely one thing nor purely another. In fact, I was constantly growing and changing, and the nature of what I was growing into was still being determined with each choice I made. John Wayne always knew who he was. I was creating myself with each breath. I could be loyal and brave, I could work hard for family, love, and community, but it would not be in the service of a truth written in stone; rather it would be in the service of a truth that could only be lived into to be understood.

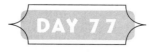

Being Right There

If we make an honest effort to feel each in-breath, then feel each out-breath, we discover why nonstealing is the next of the *yamas*. Any attempt at being present during the felt experience of a yoga pose, or sitting and breathing, brings us up against the mind's habit of stealing away from the present moment to worlds of its own creation. When we sit in the peace of a world waking up, the mind fills the silence with its habitual busyness. The *yama asteya* translates to "nonstealing," but when most of us hear this definition, we say to ourselves, "I've got that covered." And it's true, the percentage of us both practicing yoga regularly and robbing banks is low. But *asteya* is also the ability to be unconflictedly present for what is happening right now: no multitasking, no phone calls, no selfies, nothing. Just being right here for what is happening right now. And to make a beginning, we learn to pay attention to when the mind steals away.

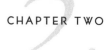

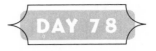

The Unconflicted Moment

One of the major challenges I face as a yoga teacher is trying to convince people to practice a behavior they have never tried because they've been too busy avoiding it. It's not like I am constantly running into students who regularly spend time resting in the felt experience of their bodies, of their breath, or of the moment but would rather be planning and worrying. The students I work with have perfected an anxious apartness from the present moment to the point where they live it on autopilot. Stealing away from the present moment just happens and happens and happens, to the point where it starts to feel like reality. The mass appeal of Eckhart Tolle's teaching and the popular phenomenon of Oprah Winfrey's meditation series with Deepak Chopra tell me that what I am observing in my yoga classes is not an isolated event. People aren't enjoying their relationship with their mind but they are not sure what to do about it.

I've found that it helps to use phrases that are both logical and inviting. Who doesn't want to be present? Who wants to feel conflicted about being here now? It also helps if I then explicitly link a yogic practice to the ability to have an unconflicted moment: "As you breathe in, know that you breathe in, and as you breathe out, know that you breathe out." It is important that I use terms that feel within reach, like "Become available to the felt experience of breathing." Then I link an approachable starting point to an approachable skill: "As we become available to the breath, in time it becomes familiar to us." This familiarity is proactive; leaving the moment is an action, staying in the moment is an action as well. Yoga turns living well into a set of small steps that lead to a series of unconflicted moments.

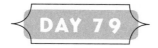

Lack

Our first attempts at present-moment awareness are like a person trying to form a word she has never heard before, or a fish trying to swim for the first time. We've explored the earth, the sea, and the skies, we've even traveled to space in search of something we never find. We've tried every conceivable virtue and vice. We've tried an infinity of cults, conspiracy theories, and time-saving devices. And all of this trying steals us away from what we are actually seeking. Yoga suggests that if we stop looking for something, we will find that it was never missing in the first place. Resting in the felt experience of being here, we realize that there is nothing lacking.

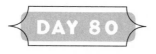

The Moment Is Complete

The form of my classes doesn't change much from year to year. This has allowed me to get better and better at the little things that make up each lesson, and as the bumps are smoothed out, more of my mental energy is freed up to look at the larger opportunities the class presents. The yoga student has set aside some time to practice life skills and the yoga teacher's job is to make that time count. We use how we are being in the body and the breath to examine how we are being in life and to practice living on

purpose. For most people, the biggest obstacle to living on purpose is the assumption that we should be afraid and live according to the logic of that fear. The fact that most students suffer the effects of some kind of trauma adds a sense of gravity to the picture. Trauma lives in the connective tissue as unfinished business, causing dis-ease throughout the mind and body. The yoga poses and the yogic breath are archetypal actions offering the student a chance to finish what has been left unfinished in her life. When she gets up off her mat and steps back into her life she knows that the moment is complete and that a new moment can begin.

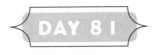

Nonstealing

Yoga doesn't just suggest that we abstain from stealing; it suggests that we explore the opposite of stealing. In my life, this means the practice of generosity. There was a period of recovery after I stopped drinking in which I was in pretty rough shape; my mind was impaired by the damage of alcohol abuse and the effects of PTSD. I had a very low tolerance for frustration and had much to grieve. After about five years of sobriety, I was ready for the demands of a path of service, a life given meaningfully to helping others with their suffering. During those five years I had developed a strong connection to my local twelve-step community, I had close friends, and I had met the woman who would become my wife. I was practicing yoga and meditation every day, so I had a pretty good handle on how to recharge my batteries and how to work through difficult emotions. Because I had learned how to give to myself, I was ready to give my whole heart to something else.

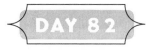

The Castle School

I flew home from the army without much of a plan beyond going to twelve-step meetings and not drinking. The counselors at my rehab had inspired me, so I spent the money I had saved while in the army on training to become an addiction counselor myself. As the training was ending, someone I knew from meetings told me about a job working with kids. I had thought I was heading into the quiet life of a counselor at a halfway house, helping people fill out job applications. What I got instead was a position working full-time with adolescents with emotional disorders.

The young people I worked with had countless different ways to ask me the same essential question: "Are you with me?" They did not want me to be smart or special; they wanted me to love the way they loved, large and sloppy, vulnerable and real. They also wanted me to be the adult, clear and calm the way they could not be, to set the boundaries they could not set. I learned to let them have the last word. I learned to be the one who said "I love you" first, to say "I'm sorry" first, to say "I forgive you" first, to say "I made a mistake" first, to meet each moment knowing that I had the real power and to use it kindly, to use that power to help them. The young people of the Castle School taught me how to be an adult, and that the essence of adulthood is generosity.

CHAPTER TWO

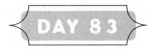

Bring a Gift

The work I did with adolescents was incredibly difficult and filled with heart-wrenching setbacks and moments that left me with no confidence or idea how I was going to meet the next day. Despite my own personal ups and downs, my role in the treatment facility was a leadership one, which meant not only was I there to implement treatment plans, I had to invent them as well. I had learned in the military that the best sort of leadership came in response to the worst sort of circumstances. I had the circumstances; now all that was needed was the leadership.

The first form of leadership I exercised was continuing my yoga practice during my lowest lows. I knew that if I was going to have a chance at leading, I would have to act like a leader even if I did not feel like one. Leaders who do yoga do yoga in good times and bad times. The second form of leadership I exercised was to continue learning. My off-hour studies were an act of faith, a vote of confidence, in myself and in my situation. A pivotal book from my education during this time was Deepak Chopra's *The Seven Spiritual Laws of Success*. In it he speaks of our ability to generate abundance in our lives through the practice of generosity. He advises us to bring a gift wherever we go, even if it is only a compliment. A turning point in my time at Castle was when I began to embrace this form of generosity and to organize my week around what gift I was bringing to the groups I was running and to the children I was counseling. By bringing a gift to my most challenging sessions, I rechanneled the energy of the situation. The Castle School was no longer happening to me; I was happening to it.

DAY 84

Holding Space

For fifteen wonderful years, the work I did at the Castle School and running yoga studios required everything I had to offer. Today I teach people to do much of what I did then. I am no longer the teacher in the room; I am the teacher's teacher. Most of the people I help never even know my name. In my years working with young people and later leading yoga studios my work was a set of actions taken. Today, my best work happens when I am doing nothing.

The first third or so of my trainings are spent getting the teachers up to speed; the rest is devoted to giving them a chance to teach, a dry run so to speak, before they take what they have learned back to their communities. It's my best work, because the teachers are learning to teach by teaching, and they are learning to teach by working together. The material of the course is presented to the group by the group itself; thirty perspectives are offered, thirty examples are given. I find the efficiency of this type of training deeply gratifying. My job during this period of the training can be summarized as "holding space." To hold space properly is to be fully present while allowing others to have their experience, to have their setbacks, and to own their victories. This is an exquisite form of generosity for me because it does not draw attention to me as the giver. Rather, it challenges me to give without the expectation of any reward other than the pleasure of seeing someone else succeed. This type of generosity is its own reward.

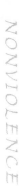
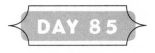

DAY 85

Silence

The final form of generosity I will be talking about is one I have learned only since becoming a father. As a young person I assumed that I would be a great dad, doing fun stuff with my kids all the time. Later, I felt I would be a great dad by laying all kinds of cool yoga wisdom on them. Once I had kids I found out that a lot of being a dad was going to get the groceries from the car and letting the dog out. There is something I do, though, that feels very important: as my children are learning through living, I am learning when to be silent and to allow them to find their own way.

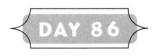

DAY 86

Flight

When we practice yoga, we are learning to live like the sun, sharing our light all day, every day, without expecting anything in return. This is an honest way of life whose essence is the spirit of generosity. However, there is a competing and natural desire for recognition that must be addressed. There is a voice that comes from deep inside us that asks, "What about me?"

When my teachers taught me the practice of loving-kindness they addressed this formally. I was taught to begin loving-kindness meditation first by offering loving-kindness to myself and then, only once I felt at peace with that practice, offering loving-kindness to others. The methodology is based on the belief that once we have learned how to love ourselves well we will have an intuitive ability to love others well. Or, more simply, that you cannot give what you do not have. This is also practical; the practice of offering loving-kindness to others is often challenging, and if we haven't learned how to recharge our batteries, our efforts at loving others well will be short-lived. Knowing how and when to take care of one's own needs precedes knowing how and when to take care of the needs of another. In the end we may be less like the sun and more like the bird that flies beneath it, learning when to flap and when to soar.

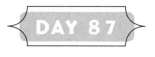

Running on Empty

An unfortunate side effect of following the path of service is that we often learn to take care of others before we have learned to take care of ourselves. We take the oath, don the uniform, and head out to serve our community, often clueless when it comes to meeting the emotional complexities of the life we have chosen. Pressures mount, cracks become gaps, and spent and without skill, we fill them with what is closest at hand. In the military it was (and, I am told, still is) alcohol, in the social work and educational fields it's food, in yoga it is a mix of eating disorders and sex. Caught up in the trap of shame, we confuse the behavior with the person and do everything except solve the problem.

The fourth *yama*, *brahmacharya* (the appropriate use of our energy), gives us a chance to talk about something people drawn to helping others don't like talking about: that we have needs too, and that failing to take care of them effectively can have dangerous consequences. I tell the teachers I train, "The good news is that it is your job to learn how to be happy."

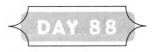

DAY 88

Brahmacharya

Brahmacharya is a call for us to practice moderation in all things but is most generally applied to sexuality. It's often misunderstood as an expectation that we be celibate, that being so will make us more enlightened; this is most definitely not its true meaning. B. K. S. Iyengar, in his discussion of *brahmacharya*, points out that the yogi Vasistha had a hundred children! To focus on celibacy is to miss the point of *brahmacharya*. It is not a call for abstinence but for temperance, to bring moderation to our thoughts, to our words, and to our deeds. The idea is that we bring mindfulness and compassion to the way we use our natural powers of attraction and seduction. It is also the idea that we learn to understand our own sexual energy and bring mindfulness and compassion to ourselves as naturally sexual beings.

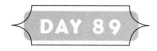

DAY 89

That Which Is Not the Self

At some point as a child I learned that I was attractive. Babysitters would tell me that I was going to be a looker. My muscles developed early and that got a lot of attention from older girls as well. At the same time, it started to seem as if certain girls had an aura of grace and beauty around them. The idea that some of them saw me the same way gave me a heady feeling. I was special when a girl thought I was special. The opposite was also true. To stop being special to someone was absolutely crushing. Caught up in life's most powerful movement, I created a self out of the ebb and flow of creation.

One of the tenets of yoga is that we think the impermanent is permanent and that which is not the self is the self. Never is this more true than when we define ourselves based on whether someone finds us "attractive." Most of us begin the practice of yoga having been lost to this confusion for some time, our relationship with our body collateral damage of the larger confusion that is human sexuality. To make a beginning with *brahmacharya* we can stand on the steady shoulders of the preceding *yamas*, holding the intention that our sexuality be nonharming, honest, and generous.

CHAPTER TWO

83

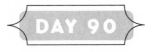

That Which Is the Self

Yoga pulls back the veil that stands between us and an integrated sense of oneness. Sitting quietly, doing nothing, we feel directly that our awareness is an aspect of the larger awareness, that our energy body is an aspect of the larger energy body, that at the level of vibration we belong to an undifferentiated larger vibration. It is an everyday event in my yoga practice to experience all of this. If I stop and get still and move from thinking to feeling, I sense directly that I am individual awareness experiencing embodiment within a universal awareness. Each time I have this experience the dramas of the separate self shift a little more from happening *to* me to happening *for* me.

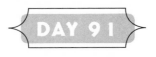

Love's List

If we are disconnected from the felt sense of who we are, it is often because we are busy relating to the story of our experience instead of having our experience. This state of affairs in yoga is called *avidya* ("spiritual ignorance") and *asmita* ("egoism" or "pride"). One is our state of disconnection, the other the mind-made self that fills the vacuum. At the heart of *avidya* is a sense that something is lacking and a craving to be whole. The acclaim that comes with high achievement can fill the void for a moment, and drugs can as well, but for most people, the thing that comes the closest to offering a taste of the divine is romantic love and sexuality. In romantic love and in the timelessness of sex we experience the moment in all its depth and wonder. These moments tell us that we are hardwired for timeless bliss. Romantic love and sexuality are doorways into an aspect of ourselves that deserves significant investigation. Yoga provides that investigation and provides us with some important perspectives on romantic love and sexuality. But before we go into that, I feel it's only fair to list some of the things romantic love and sexuality tell us about ourselves: Love's List.

We have a vast capacity for love; our favorite activity is to appreciate someone; opposites attract; timelessness is our favorite time; vanishing into a moment feels like coming home; our bodies are divinely competent; we have a genius for giving and receiving love; no motivation available to us matches the power of love.

Namo nama, I bow, I bow to the perfect energy of love.

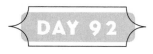

Life's List

Although love is definitely the most potent experience available to us in ordinary consciousness, there are a number of flow states that we enter into on a regular basis, giving us a glimpse into life outside of time and self. Sports, art, music, gardening, cooking, cleaning (I like to iron shirts), dancing, waiting tables—in short, anything people are willing to practice regularly offers us a timeless flow state outside of the grind of psychological time. An examination of life's list of flow states begs the question, why aren't we doing this all the time?

If we can flow into cooking and cleaning, standing and walking, sitting and breathing, why don't we? We can and do; it's called yoga. *Brahmacharya* is not saying that we should place sexuality above or below any other action we take in life; it is saying that it has a time and a place, just like almost everything else. The time and place for timelessness, however, is always now. We have within ourselves the ability to give ourselves to whatever the moment brings the same way we give ourselves to one another in love. Yoga is a way to cultivate that ability.

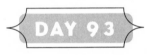

The Deliberate Use of Our Energy

The last twenty years of my life have seen a dramatic increase in the scope of my responsibilities. At thirty I was a student and a waiter living in a low-rent apartment with two other young men. My possessions amounted to a futon, a comfy chair, a CD player, and a bike. I was single, and although I felt accountable to a good handful of friends and colleagues, I was responsible for myself and myself alone. As the years unfolded I found myself in a permanent position of authority in an ever-increasing circle of highly complex relationships. Not only was I in a position of authority in the field of yoga, it was an emerging field, so I, and those around me, were shepherding a whole

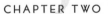

new possibility into the world. Many of the pioneers who brought modern yoga to the four corners of the globe were my contemporaries, talking with me about a dream they had one day, then creating massive movements the next. I was literally present at the birth of modern yoga. It was a big deal. Within just a few years it became clear to me that who I was and what I did mattered. What I could create and what I could inspire would rest largely on how I lived my life.

I understood that my life was a container for divine energy and that if it had strong boundaries, then an intense flow of energy could pass through it without doing me or anyone else harm. Strong boundaries also give me the ability to direct and modulate the energy that moves through me so that it is used in the service of the highest good. The *yamas* are the means by which I build my container, and nowhere has that been more important than the integrity with which I use my sexual energy. How I use my energy as a leader answers the question every student has in the back of her mind: "Are you trying to serve God, or are you trying to be God?" The answer matters.

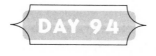

Your Love Will Be Safe with Me

There is a song by the group Bon Iver that I have been listening to over the last few months. One morning, even though I'd heard the song a hundred times or so, I finally made out the last line: "Your love will be safe with me." This line captures my intention for how I want to relate to the people in my life, specifically around matters of the heart and sexuality. I want to be an

CHAPTER TWO

ally, to stand next to the people in my life. To help shoulder their burden as they attempt to meet life with open hearts. I want their love to be safe with me. I want them to know that I will support them as they try to be true to the loves in their lives and as they try to use their sexual energy wisely. I can think of no better definition, expression, or affirmation of *brahmacharya* than "Your love will be safe with me."

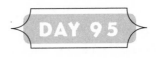

The End of Craving

Brahmacharya is a complex practice of balancing discipline and freedom, wisdom and compassion. We make a beginning by standing firm in the intention that our sexuality be nonharming, honest, and generous. We continue this work by looking at the final *yama*, *aparigraha*, which deconstructs the logic of fear by advocating "nonpossessiveness" or "nonhoarding." *Aparigraha* can be applied to our attachment to our thoughts, to our beliefs and relationships, and to our desires. *Aparigraha* brings mindfulness and compassion to the experience of wanting something—and the fear of losing it.

Because of the intensity of the feelings generated by fear and desire, yoga guides us to set aside time to sit with these feelings without judging or trying to change them. The process of mindfulness seeks only to know what is true. Sitting with the sort of intense craving sexual desire creates, one notices the desire to seek an end of craving by gratifying it. A married friend of mine once said of a man she was attracted to, "Maybe I should just sleep with him and see if there is anything there." When you are at the height of a craving, it's not the time to make a major life decision. If we are willing to sit with these feelings a little longer, we find that they begin to fade and then pass altogether. We find the end of craving by doing nothing. Then, when the craving returns, we have the opportunity to know life by being with it, seeking only to know what is true. Sitting quietly doing nothing, wisdom comes and compassion grows all by itself.

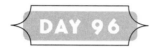

More Than This

Greed and sexual misconduct go hand in hand, and neither has a high approval rating. Because of the shame we feel about sexual misconduct and the confused state that precedes it, we tend not to get around to talking about this aspect of our lives, let alone working with it. The demands of my personal aspirations require that I pay attention, however. I made clear commitments to being a husband, a yoga teacher, and, eventually, a father. In each instance these commitments brought a light into my life with which to get to know my own shadow. What I can say about my own personal and professional work is that it comes down to which version of myself I want to invest in. There is a version of myself who needs more than this, and there is a version of myself who can be more because of this.

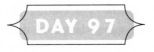

Creation and Limitation

To manifest anything we must accept limitation.

Anodea Judith

While *aparigraha* does include sexual craving, it primarily speaks to our everyday desires for food, shelter, social position, and control over our environment. It is an absolutely perfect arena for the practice of yoga because it takes place right where we live, in the everyday scramble to make a life for ourselves in the shared space we call our town, our city, our country, our planet. We tend to seek solutions that involve movement, and we tend to seek solutions that involve more. *Aparigraha* is the practice of training ourselves to see the opportunity in less, the opportunity in space, the opportunity in stillness and allowing. It is the sense of when to accept limitation as the first step in creation.

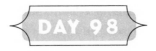

Rob Machado

Rob Machado was one of the best surfers of his generation. He surfed professionally for many years and is now a sponsored rep for one of the big clothing lines, traveling the world surfing and promoting corporate surfing togs, as well as helping people in need get access to clean water. I often settle my mind and lift my spirits by watching footage of him surfing endless lefts in Indonesia. In one of my favorite videos, there is a wave that he catches that looks as if it goes on for several hundred yards. The camera is on a helicopter, so we can watch the wave forming over and over again and Rob's intuitive flow across its endless sections. He is in perfect harmony with the wave's utter imperfection. Watching Rob surf, I learned that art begins, like creation, with limitation. We train year after year to perfect our skills, but art doesn't happen until those skills meet the need to improvise. Art doesn't happen until life does.

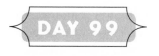

An Appropriate Response

It is difficult to find fault with the desires for safety, food, and shelter. They seem like the appropriate response to having a body. In fact, *aparigraha* is the practice of an appropriate response to embodiment. It is acting in the awareness that anything we are or possess on the physical plane is impermanent. It is acting in the awareness that we are part of an infinite web of interdependence and anything we need, or will need, will be delivered to us, not by our efforts at control but by this infinite web. It is acting in the knowledge that anything we do to any part of the web of interdependence is something we are doing to ourselves. The Bible states, "Whatsoever you do to the least of my brothers that you do unto me also." Carrying this awareness into each choice we make is *aparigraha*.

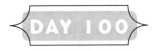

Managing the Unmanageable

When I walk into a room to teach a class there is a pleasant sort of anarchy presiding over the space. If I want to begin class on time I can try to manage the unmanageable by going to each person and forcing her to get to her mat, or I can align with the flow of life by practicing the *yamas*. I choose the latter and simply ask people to take a comfortable seat. This works every time. It is nonviolent because I am not attempting to take away the students' right to choose. It is honest because I am making the simple, straightforward statement that class has begun. It is generous because it is motivated by the desire to begin and end the class on time, fulfilling the agreement I have made with my students. It is an appropriate use of my energy because I am not drawing undue attention to myself. And it is an exercise in *aparigraha* because I am acknowledging that *I* will not begin the class, *we* will.

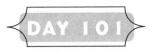

Racquetball

Throughout college and my years in the army, I practiced racquetball in much the same way I would later practice yoga: I made a study of it. Toward the end of this time I was watching two advanced players. The younger one was rushing about. The older one seemed to play with very little effort. He just took three steps, then hit the ball, three steps, three steps. The older gentleman was winning every point despite the effort the younger man was exerting. Although I was also very young at the time, it was still clear to me that the junior player thought he had to make the game happen and the older man knew the game was already happening. He simply needed to find his place in it. Later I would find this same basic wisdom in the *yamas*.

THREE WAYS TO PRACTICE NONVIOLENCE

1) Practice self-care like everything else depends on it.
2) Make a commitment to do no harm.
3) Practice kindness, honesty, and generosity all of the time, everywhere, in every circumstance.

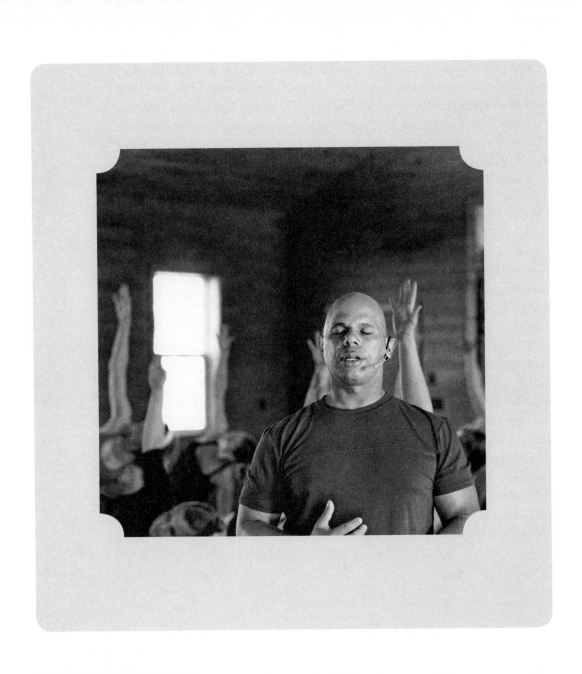

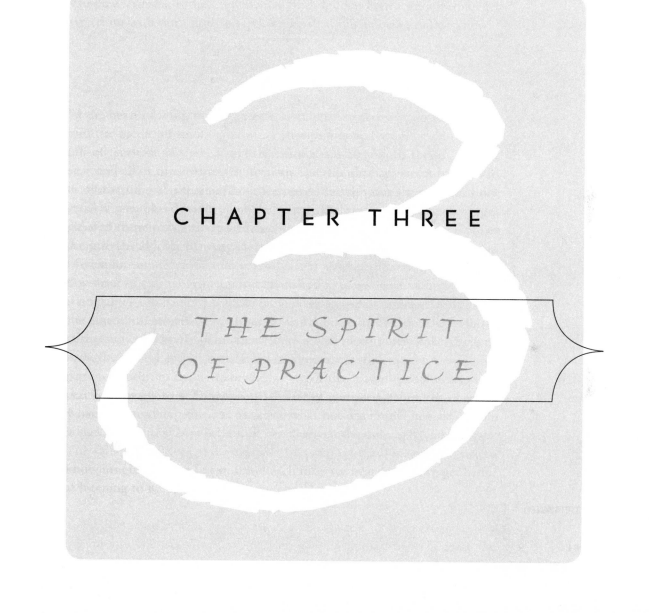

CHAPTER THREE

THE SPIRIT
OF PRACTICE

Yoga is not a *having* practice; it is a *being* practice. The difference matters. I spent my time in the military in the army, and our mission was to take and hold ground. That was definitely a having practice. Later, I worked delivering packages, and that too was a having practice. Our clients were not interested in being a package; theirs was the desire to have, and to have whatever it was they were waiting for yesterday. Having practices are finite. The package arrives, the manifest is signed, and the moment is over. Having begins and ends. Being is timeless. Being practices are in a process of continual unfolding. They never end. Sustainability and momentum in a being practice are coequal partners with whatever action is being practiced. In yoga, the limb of sustainability and momentum is the *niyamas*, the habits that lead to success on the spiritual path. I teach this limb as the work we do to cultivate the spirit of practice.

We can think of the *yamas* as a set of boundaries that prevent us from falling into low-vibration patterns like greed and ill will and encourage us to practice high-vibration ones like honesty and generosity. The *yamas* bring our attention to patterns or habits that will not serve us; the *niyamas* focus our attention on habits that will. We cannot run marathons without habits and practices that deliver a high state of fitness. In yoga the cultivation of happiness and freedom works the same way. The *niyamas* are an explicit set of practices to help us establish and maintain the happiness and freedom we seek year in and year out.

Like attracts like, and when we are in low-vibration patterns the world seems to be with us. When I was drinking I had no idea how few people actually drank the way I did. It seemed like the whole world thought everything was better with a glass in hand. The same is true as we take up high-vibration practices. Before long our friends, our partner, our colleagues, our communities form part of an extended web of support helping us to choose and sustain a life that expresses happiness and freedom.

The *niyamas* are comprehensive, bringing mindfulness and compassion into five overlapping aspects of our lives. These are *sauca* ("purity"), *santosa* ("contentment"), *tapas* ("zeal" or "austerity"), *svadhyaya* ("self-study"), and *isvara-pranidhana* ("devotion to a higher power"). Each of these five observances keeps us aligned with our true selves. Any one of the *niyamas* could be the practice of a lifetime. *Santosa*, the practice of contentment, for example, is the willingness to work with things as they are. The relevance of this practice is universal, as are the challenges to its successful implementation.

My teachers tell me to let the moment come to me, and I encourage you to do the same. To practice any of the *yamas* or *niyamas* you must eventually practice all of them, so let the moment dictate which *niyama* you are focusing on. That being said, once you choose to focus on a *niyama*, stay with it for a while. These practices shed light on aspects of our lives that we have kept in the shadows, and those shadows will not give up their secrets to a match struck, creating a momentary light. To get where the *niyamas* can take us we will need to turn on a light and keep it on. This chapter is dedicated to turning on a light and the heart that chooses to do so.

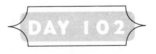

Freedom

The *yamas* and *niyamas* are a set of healthy self-boundaries and practices that sustain and maintain our freedom. Within any victim narrative, freedom is something that must be gained. The assumption of the *yamas* and the *niyamas* is that we are already free and that we maintain our freedom by binding ourselves to love in all its forms. This might sound like a pretty big project, but we don't have to do it all at once; we just have to do it now

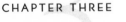

with whatever the moment brings. We just have to do the next right thing. And if we keep it that simple, love will be there and we will find ourselves free to choose it.

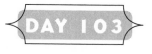

Sauca

The first *niyama* is *sauca*, or purity, of the mind and the body. It encompasses all that we give and all that we receive, and it is the ultimate sustainability and momentum tool. I recently embarked on a food routine designed to help boost my *sauca*. Three days into eating high-energy foods in appropriate quantities I went for a hike and felt like I was twenty-five. The practice of *sauca* delivers in such an impactful manner that it is surprising that we have not made it the entirety of yoga. Consider what happens when we clean up a room or a yard, when we clean and iron a shirt, or when we treat our loved ones kindly for a weekend. Treat anything with a little love and care and it blooms like a flower in spring. *Sauca* is the art of love and care.

CHAPTER THREE

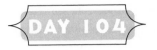

All We Receive

My Buddhist teachers have taught me the concept of right consumption. They have encouraged me to make a study of the food I eat, the books I read, and the conversations I participate in and to examine the effect allowing this food, this thought, this emotion into my mind-body has upon my state of consciousness. Is binge-watching *Homeland* really making my life better? How does it feel after I have a meatball sub for lunch? Which foods, relationships, and activities bring a sense of happiness and freedom and which don't?

Right consumption is a straightforward way for me to move through the world as an adult taking responsibility for how I am voting with my feet, my words, my wallet. The practice of right consumption, like any other skillful practice, brings a light into the areas of my life that have been in the shadows of habit. It offers me a right-sized sense of the impact of my choices and a chance to check in with my heart before I make a decision. When we are new to the practice, it can also be an opportunity to judge ourselves and others harshly. This is why compassion is a coequal partner with mindfulness. Since yoga is ultimately the alignment of one's values with one's actions, right consumption is the perfect place to start. For me, this means understanding what we are worthy of receiving. As you pause in the moment before you do or do not allow yourself to receive something, start to bring your attention to the emotional body. What do you think you deserve?

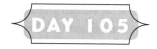

Good Orderly Direction

Twelve-step programs are sensitive to the fact that the word "God" and the concept of a higher power mean something different to everyone. The literature and the ongoing dialogue within the meetings avoid assumptions about an individual's belief. As a result, many of the people who have been successful in what is an overtly spiritual program of recovery from addiction have been agnostics or atheists. Some turn the word "God" into an acronym that stands for "good orderly direction." *Sauca* is good orderly direction in action.

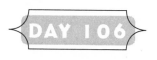

Sauca as Generosity

When I began working with children, one of the rules of thumb I was taught was that while you can't control the kids, you can control the environment. Research indicates that children feel calmer and behave better if their environment feels good, orderly, and directed. This brought my attention to the impact our environment has on our inner life. At work I made every effort to provide the children I cared for with a good orderly environment and with a process that felt fair and transparent. How I applied the rules, offered words of encouragement, and made decisions in general were

CHAPTER THREE

intended to project the sense that everyone was being treated fairly, always. In my practice I create order around my mat and my cushion. As a student and participant in the various communities I am a part of, I keep in mind that I am sharing a space, whether it is a yoga classroom or the parking lot at a local surf spot. I know that I can express loving-kindness toward the other individuals in my community by acting in ways that support calm, clean order without judging those who do not. The final frontier in my own practice has been to bring this same intention to the space I create for myself.

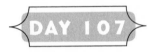

Purity of Purpose

As someone who started life in an orphanage I have found it hard to get close to people in authority and have had to be content to watch from afar. Since I was raised by nuns, men in authority have been particularly hard to connect with. Instead of talking to my male role models, I had to study how they lived and have developed the ability to study in detail. I know all the stats and the blood, sweat, and tears behind the numbers. When this person won his first championship and when he won his last. How this person moves his shoulder before throwing a pass and the moment I knew that person's cutback was world-class. The calm he displayed while writing orders in battle, the calm he displayed while going to jail for civil rights, and the calm he displayed walking up the stairs of a burning tower. Watching from afar has given me the ability to see what those closer may not catch or value, because they can see all the flaws.

Every day I carry the examples of these role models in my heart, and I never feel as if I am meeting a moment alone because of the wealth of courage they have shown in circumstances almost always more difficult than the ones I have found myself in. Each generation educates the next, and I have been told that to teach is to demonstrate. What all of these men have demonstrated is a purity of purpose that stirred their hearts and allowed them to rise above their circumstances to express something meaningful about the human spirit.

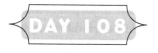

DAY 108

Clarity

A metaphor for *sauca* is that it's like finding something lost in a room that is clean and orderly as opposed to finding something that is lost in a room that is messy. The role *sauca* plays in our practice is both practical and deeply metaphysical. On a practical level, a clean house and healthy diet make getting to our mat and to our cushion easier and more enjoyable. On a metaphysical level, *sauca* prepares our hearts and minds for yoga.

Most of us come to yoga in an existential muddle. We've been living in a civilization whose narrative has been co-opted by the belief that our economy must grow or die. Our duty to the collective is to consume and to help others consume. Within the first few minutes of meeting someone, we ask the question we have all learned to ask: "What do you do?" In the world we have created for ourselves what someone does for work pretty much sums them up. The distinctions between doing, having, and being have become unavailable to us when formulating a vision of the good life.

Our inner life has gone untended as we have sought to find happiness without it. The first few years in yoga are understandably somewhat confused. We are like amnesia victims, only what we have forgotten is not who we are but what matters. The tenets of yoga amount to actions that can be taken to clean up our inner life. As we do so, we discover a heart here, a mind there, and, eventually, a purpose.

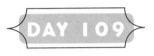

The Altar of the Mind

As I was contemplating ordering some fried chicken in the prepared foods section at my local supermarket, a friend of mine came up to me and asked me, "What are you putting in that temple?" His appearance in that moment felt both divinely inspired and deeply unwelcome. I was young and fit and had not had to work that hard to become so. My friend was older and was a bodyworker who'd had to give some thought to how he was treating himself. As I turned to look at him I noticed how fit and strong he was. In an inelegant yet helpful turn of phrase, yoga calls the body the "food sheath," which helps me to remember that my body is literally made out of whatever I eat. And if the body is the temple, the mind is the altar of that temple. What I eat is what my body is composed of, and what I place on the altar of my mind determines what my world is composed of. This can feel like a lot of responsibility, and I did not like my friend's reminding me of that responsibility. Yoga softens the blow by reminding us that mastery of a practice like *sauca* happens by degrees. We only need to be willing to do the next right thing.

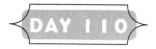

DAY 110

What We Give

The concepts of charity and loving-kindness can be found in the teachings of both Jesus Christ and the Buddha, and they constitute the manner in which the founders of two of humanity's most enduring religions thought we should relate to one another. The definitions of these words are, for all intents and purposes, exactly the same. They are that one who would practice Christianity or Buddhism should learn to love her neighbor as herself (this argument is in the Yoga Sutras, too—1.33). *Sauca* offers us the opportunity to practice this sort of kindness in our everyday interactions, purifying what we habitually give the way we are purifying what we habitually receive. The idea is that acting with generosity toward others is not a chore but rather an opportunity to begin living really well. Being kind feels great, has a high probability of being well received, and rarely leads to regret. I would also like to add that as a husband, father, friend, son, brother, teacher, and business owner, choosing kindness always seems to get me where I want to go. It's pleasant, life affirming, and practical all at the same time.

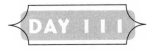

The Earth Beneath Our Feet

There is something absolutely magical and mysterious about being here now. Why here, why now, why me? If we look down we see Earth spinning on its axis beneath our feet. If we look up we catch a glimpse of infinity, the stars, the sun, the moon, for company in a timeless moment in a timeless eternity. When we look into the eyes of another living being we see our own awareness looking back. *Sauca* asks, "What do we need with more?" It invites us to be just here, to look just here, to see the beauty all around us. It tells us to be the beauty we see all around us, to choose the beauty and the love it reflects. To breathe that beauty in, then breathe that beauty out. To let our life be nothing but that. To stand strong and at peace with the earth beneath our feet, breathing life in, breathing life out, and letting go of everything else.

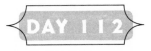

Something That Has Been Lost

Yoga does not give us a new Earth, a new spring, a new birth, a new death, a new now; it gives us eyes to see what has always been. The food I eat reflects who I believe myself to be. My family's traumas and stories around food, my culture's traumas and stories around food, have replaced my own understanding. I see the stories, I feel the traumas, feel the victories, feeling what it was to emerge from depression into unlimited abundance. I feed the stories; I nourish the trauma, I clean my plate. Ten years of "making weight" in wrestling and months on almost no food in ranger training remind me of what it is to want and how it is better not to. A friend recommends I keep it simple: Eat no more than two or three different kinds of food per meal. Keep the meals moderate and eat every few hours. Drink a lot of water. I say okay. As the days go by I begin to see that my body isn't a story or a trauma. It feels the pain of my ancestors, it feels the pain of my own life, but it is not that pain. I see what has always been.

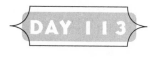

Contentment

As you can probably imagine, my early years on my mat were a big deal. Everything that I had been learning about life in sobriety was confirmed and affirmed in a magnificent way by the practices and teachings of yoga. I went after the practice of asana with all I had. I studied the forms and rituals, practiced at four in the morning by candlelight, and felt the power of an ancient way of life living through me.

Then I went to my first hot vigorous yoga class. If yoga had seemed like an awesome church, this seemed like a mediocre gym. I was sweating a lot, which made finding my footing in a wide-legged forward bend difficult. I had to put more emphasis on my upper body to maintain my stability. I paused, then shrugged. Sometimes your mat is slippery and sometimes it's not. Sometimes yoga happens in an awesome church, sometimes it happens in a mediocre gym. Contentment is the practice of succeeding no matter what.

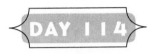

Santosa

After writing about the power of love and the power of purity it seems like contentment—the second of the *niyamas, santosa*—might be a little underwhelming. Then you look at what it really is and you begin to think, "Maybe contentment is the key to life?" The willingness to work with things as they are feels like the start of everything. Can we be content to work with the family that we have, the health that we have, the time that we have, the body that we have, the mental and emotional state that we are in, the money that we have, the challenges that we have, the moment that we are in? This feels like the ultimate skill, to see the opportunity in whatever the moment brings and to begin there.

Yoga would say that you don't have to be perfect at it to get started. It helps to reflect on how many times you have thought a situation was all bad only to discover numerous opportunities and blessings within that same situation. It is also helpful to reflect on the rational observation that we have no other choice than to work with things as they are, so we might as well get good at it. I find inspiration whenever I remember all of the leaders through the ages who found themselves in an impossible situation and chose to create something positive anyway. However we arrive at it, *santosa* offers us the opportunity to take what is and to create something beautiful with it.

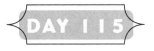

When to Begin

I made a friend in high school; he was a year younger than I was, so we were not as close in school as we would later become in our twenties and thirties. We shared the odd sadness of the adopted and a passion for natural beauty. He was a consummate woodsman, having gone through rigorous training in Alaska and the Rockies with the National Outdoor Leadership School, and could pass on what he had learned without seeming to try. My friend, Jude, taught me to love silence, the forests of northern Maine, and the period of consideration as someone examines the water before fishing. The eye starts with the basic flow of the river: where it runs deep, where it runs shallow, where it runs fast, and where it runs slow or circles back; what parts are shaded and how the movement of the sun will affect the light on the water. Then there is the riverbed itself: sand, mud, vegetation, pebbles, rocks, and boulders are taken into account, and what kind of wildlife likes each. Next is the ecosystem that has grown up around this stretch of river. Who lives here and what are they up to when? Jude watched to see what insects were hatching and how that was playing out. Were they emerging within the river itself, were they coming to the surface and staying there, or were they leaving the river altogether, taking flight at the beginning of an

entirely new existence? Was there something else the fish were feeding on? Were the fish bottom-feeders, or did they spy food on the surface and take athletic leaps, rising into the air? We fished a river in Canada for a couple of weeks when the salmon were not feeding at all. We assessed the river in silence, feeling for the moment when we were content to choose the lure we would use that day and make a beginning.

Rest in peace, my dear friend; you are missed.

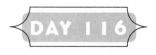

When to Keep Going

I was taught land navigation before the widespread adoption of GPS. The technology of the time was a map and a compass. In the military, they would take you out into the woods and tell you to find several consecutive points over the course of a couple of hours. Each point was about eight football fields from the last, through Georgia pine forest. Before you began you would find your pace count by walking one hundred yards and counting how many steps it took you. My count was sixty-four paces. You would determine your direction with your compass and head out, counting paces as you went. If you were wise you would recheck your direction every fifty yards or so. The direction your compass provided was usually good enough so that the decisive factor in determining the location of the checkpoint you were seeking was the pace count. New students would get anxious about 80 percent of the way there, unconsciously shortening their steps as they began looking around for the checkpoint. Because of this change, your pace count would lead you to think the checkpoint should be located about

10 percent short of your actual destination. This precipitated a crisis during which the student would stop using her navigation skills and start frantically (and uselessly) looking around for the checkpoint. It took me between five and ten attempts to figure out what was going on. Eventually, I learned when to be content with my direction and keep going.

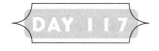

When to Let Go

There is a full-sized bronze statue of a whale at the natural history museum in Santa Cruz, California, where I live with my family. When we first moved there my daughter, Jasmine, was five years old. The whale was the sort of thing families with children that age gravitate to, and within days of our arrival on the West Coast we were at the natural history museum, running about its grassy front yard and climbing upon its very awesome bronze whale. After a period of gazing at the whale and touching the whale Jasmine began climbing on it. Her father was already prepared for this so that when she needed a hand, a hand was there. She walked up the tail, then onto the whale's back. When she got to the highest point I had two options: I could let her go and know that if she fell away from me there was nothing I could do about it, or I could stop the exploration. There was a pause, and then I let go, content to let her take life's hand. She walked to the head of the whale and jumped off, never knowing the courage and faith it took for me to be her dad.

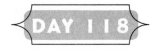

When to Speak

My neighbor lost his house this year. He is a contractor and just did not get enough work. I did not know of his troubles until I came home to find him moving out. There was enough ambiguity around what was happening that I could have gone into my house and avoided an unpleasant situation. My wife was with me, and as she was getting out of the car, I paused. My first spiritual community was a twelve-step program, and it saves lives by not being afraid of other people's pain. I reflected. My yoga community is informed by the principles of loving-kindness and compassion, which guide us as we work with other people's pain. I understood. My years as a counselor and as a yoga teacher have taught me that people are afraid of being rejected for being imperfect, for having pain. I acted. I told my wife I would be inside in a minute and got out of the car. I walked over to where my neighbor was moving his belongings out of the house he had hoped to raise his children in, content to say, "Thank you for being my neighbor," to share his pain, and to say good-bye.

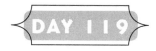

When to Be Silent

I taught a four P.M. class on Tuesdays and Thursdays for several years. I loved that class because my students seemed thrilled to get out of work, get in a yoga class, and, at five thirty, still have the rest of the evening free. There was a young man who came regularly. He could do the entire class with relative ease but felt it necessary to do everything one breath behind. If I was inhaling up, he was exhaling down. He did this for ninety minutes twice a week for at least two years. It drove me crazy. From long practice teaching I have a rule I impose on myself: if a student is not harming herself, another student, or the process, I leave her alone. I impose this rule on myself to safeguard the student's access to yoga. Day after day I was content to leave him be and work with my reaction to him, learning to teach through a little discomfort. I left that studio and left Boston, coming back once in a while to visit family and for work. When I was sitting at a juice bar on one of these visits, this same young man came up to me and thanked me for his years in class. He said he had been going through a very difficult time, the very same sort of hard time I was going through at that moment, in fact, and that his time in class with me had made a huge difference. We smiled and laughed together and when he was gone I was content to have been silent.

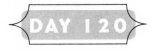

When to Say Thank You

I have a prayer that I use to access *santosa*. It is the simple statement "Thank you for bringing me here." I began using it each time I took my seat at a twelve-step meeting. The prayer felt like sanity. Then it started showing up everywhere. I would say it stopping on a hike through a forest. I would say it at the beginning of a yoga class, in the middle when the students were in tree pose, at the end while they were in *savasana*. I say it now at bedtime lying quietly next to my children, being the calm presence that helps them go to sleep. I say it looking back at the California coastline, sitting on my surfboard. I say it when the teachers I teach are leading a class and I can see how each generation makes way for the next. These days I am saying it everywhere I go and it is more than enough. There is nothing to be added or subtracted; I am content to say thank you.

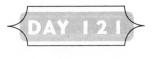

Tapas

I am a warrior from a warrior people. All the brown men I saw on television growing up were warriors, and there was no question in my mind when I stepped out onto a playing field or a wrestling mat that I had been born to bring it. I did not feel any connection to desks and chalkboards and simply bided my time in the classroom until I could get to practice or, better yet, an actual contest complete with uniforms, timers, a scoreboard, consequences, and a chance to do my best. Later, I discovered all the other ways my peers do their best. Some make music, others money; some write screenplays, still others write computer code. Where I live people ride fifty-foot waves, and each generation quite a few of us find our calling as parents. Almost all of us have found something that calls to us across eternity to be great, to be unstoppable. "*Tapas*" is the name for that special fire that rises up in us when we decide to do our best.

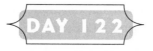

No Guarantees

I was recently talking to a young person of significant promise who struggles with addiction. He had previously tried not drinking and had managed to go six months before relapsing. He was now three months sober and trying twelve-step meetings for the first time, which he said was helping. I told him that the hand he had been dealt when it came to drinking was a poor one, but the hand he had been dealt when it came to sobriety was an amazing one. That he should be very excited about what sobriety had in store for him, with one stipulation: that he treat this opportunity as the only one he knew he was going to get. I asked my young friend to understand this one thing: the chance he had now was the best one anyone could ever hope for, but that there were no guarantees of another one coming his way. I told him to live this chance for all he was worth. To leave it all on the field this time, every ounce of himself. I told him to practice sobriety with *tapas*.

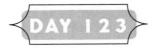

Every Day

As a young man my thoughts were molded by the movies I watched and the television shows that were my first addiction. In these depictions of life there was always a defining moment where the hero won the day and resolved all his issues. My time as an athlete did not exactly confirm this representation, in that it took many ordinary moments in practice to make one extraordinary moment in competition, but at least resolution was available within the span of a season. In my twenties, I woke up from the hell realm of active addiction to discover that every day was a playing field on which a truly defining moment was taking place. Not only did it "matter" to the self-help books I was reading how I lived each moment of each day, it mattered to *me*. After years of rationalization and justification, I realized that I actually hated ducking a punch. I hated being too lost in a pattern to meet the moment honestly. I hated letting others down. I hated letting myself down. I wanted to practice life the way I had once wanted to practice sports. I wanted to live with wisdom and heart. I wanted to live as if I knew that every day matters. I understood what *tapas* was long before I had ever heard the word, and after many years working with all kinds of people I think we all do.

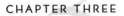

CHAPTER THREE

116

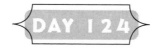

How Often Do I Practice?

Q. How often should I meditate?

A. You should meditate every day until you want to meditate every day. Then you should do what you want.

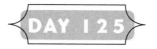

When Do I Practice?

I find it wise to keep in mind the fact that I am practicing for a reason. That there will be a moment when I can make a choice out of my conditioned reactivity or I can make a choice that I have practiced, a choice that reflects my highest aspirations, my core values and beliefs. And I have come to understand that it will matter to me and those I love which choice I make. We practice in good times so that we will have the momentum to practice in the bad ones. We practice when it is easy so that we will practice when it is hard. We practice in a safe, controlled setting so when it is scary and uncertain we will know what to do. We practice in the light what we wish to remember in the dark.

CHAPTER THREE

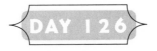

Catching the Ball

There is a story I use to illustrate the connection between practicing yoga and meeting adversity. When I was in tenth grade, I made the varsity football team but I was still a little small, so they made me a wide receiver. I ran pass patterns day after day in practice, and during the first quarter of my first game I did a lot of the same without getting passed to. At some point in the second quarter, right about the time I had come to the belief that football was really just running on beautifully manicured fields in the sun, a shadow emerged from the backfield; it was the ball—and it was coming to me! Adrenaline pumped through me so hard I literally leaped into the air. I turned and ran toward the ball, only to have it fly over my head. The walk back to the huddle was hard; our quarterback was one of the best in the league, it was his last year, and I had let him down. The rest of my team wasn't very happy either. The pain of my failure helped me to pay attention and to learn. Two things had to be remembered. When the ball is thrown to you it's not like in practice; you feel different, but that mustn't change the way you behave. My quarterback had passed the ball according to the patterns we had practiced and the trajectory I was on before I saw the ball was coming to me. If I wanted to catch the ball next time I had to run the pattern the way we had practiced. The stakes would be higher, my heart would be pumping pure adrenaline, but all I needed to do was stay on course. That season I made several memorable receptions, and each time I just ran my pattern.

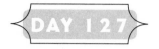

How Do We Practice When Things Are Hard?

When I was in my twenties I did not have a family or a career and I had the profound good health of the young, so I had to learn about practicing through the hard times by watching other people's examples. What I saw was that we all have the ability to stay true to ourselves, and our beliefs, in the face of life's greatest challenges. It just takes a lot of hard work before-hand. I saw people meet terminal illness, divorce, and loss with faith and grace, and in every instance they had strong spiritual practices that only got stronger when they needed them to. I saw the ball called "meeting adversity with grace and grit" thrown to members of my community over and over again. I watched in awe as they ran their pattern and made the catch. The first lesson I drew from this is that you don't get thrown the ball every play, but when you do, you want to be ready to catch it. The second lesson is that when someone on your team catches the ball, it really matters. Everyone is stronger in their faith and in their practice when someone catches the ball. The third lesson was that I knew what I wanted to give back to my community when the ball came my way; I knew who I wanted to be in the lives of those who watched and cared as I met adversity. I wanted to offer yet another example of spiritual practice working when it matters the most. This would require skill and perseverance but most of all it would require courage. Courage is a fire in our hearts, a fire we stoke with *tapas*.

CHAPTER THREE

3

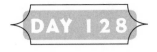

Carpe Diem

Looking over the first three *niyamas*—*sauca* ("purity"), *santosa* ("contentment"), and *tapas* ("zeal" or "austerity")—we see a plan for sustainability and momentum emerging. Whether we are running a marathon or running a restaurant, we are setting ourselves up for success by bringing love and care to both our inner environment and to our outer one. When I think of *sauca* I think of waking up to a clean, quiet house feeling inspired physically, emotionally, and mentally. *Santosa* provides us with a clear commitment to playing the hand we have been dealt without regret. At this point *tapas* is pretty much a done deal. We are in alignment with life on life's terms and we are bringing our A game. *Tapas* adds the quality of insight. We know the value of this moment and are awake to the blessing that is called seizing the day.

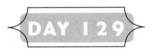

Self-study

Some of us get to wake up to yoga gradually. A doctor recommends acupuncture or a yoga class. We start showing up and over time are drawn into a life that works from the inside out. Others get thrown into the deep end

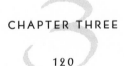

and have no choice but to learn to swim. Cancer and addiction tend to do that to people; addiction certainly did it for me. For other people, self-study arrives slowly but surely. For those of us brought to the brink of death by our lifestyle choices, self-study begins right away. In either case, it starts when we can honestly say that we do not know.

It seems a simple enough thing to say, but really it's the hardest part of coming to yoga. If we can admit that we do not know something, then we can learn anything. If we cannot admit that we do not know, we will remain blind to what we could learn. I think we are afraid to say "I don't know" because we think in terms of black and white. Either I say I know and I retain the power of choice, or I say I do not know and I give my power away. In this scenario, retaining choice seems preferable even if it is at the expense of remaining stuck in a life that does not work. What yoga offers is another option, one in which learning does not degrade the learner, nor does it take away her power of choice. In yoga, learning happens by degrees, and each degree is another turning point in the student's life, another moment of choice.

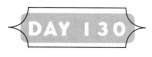

Beginning at the Beginning

Self-study, or *svadhyaya*, is the fourth *niyama*. It comes after we have been asked to cultivate a lot of simple habits that turn out to be challenging to acquire. We find that these practices go against the grain of our individual and collective sense of self, that what stands between us and an act of kindness, or honesty, is not race, or gender, or politics, but just plain old-fashioned self-protection. We may mutter unkind stereotypes under our breath, but it is not because we are fundamentally against any particular group of people. What we discover is that we are against any threat to the immediate gratification of the self. Any honest effort at the preceding *yamas* and *niyamas* reveals that our behavior reflects our self-definition and that that definition has gone largely unchecked and unexamined for as long as we can remember. *Svadhyaya* suggests that we are ready to begin at the beginning, with the self that we are protecting, and to see if it is indeed worth all the effort. It suggests that we do not have to do so alone, that in fact it is focusing purely on ourselves that got us into this mess in the first place. *Svadhyaya* is not only the invitation to become self-aware, it is the practice of learning from those who have gone down the path of self-awareness before us.

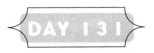

A Private Courage

I have witnessed many different kinds of courage. The courage in a locker room before a football game; the courage of my oldest sibling, Wendy, and my oldest child, Jasmine, the first through the door, always; the courage of my parents going to work day after day to provide for their children; the courage in a room full of addicts in the final stages of their addiction, giving life another try; the courage of a room full of people meditating for weeks at a time in an effort to meet life honestly; the courage of my father-in-law as he has gone through the crucible of cancer treatment and the years that followed; the courage of a couple walking down the aisle to pledge their lives to each other; the courage of a pregnant mother as she awaits the pains and trials of giving birth; the courage with which parents work to give their children a better world than the one they have known; the courage of the public school teacher; and the courage of the nurses, the doctors, the police and fire personnel of every town or city I have ever lived in. There is the courage of young people as they take their first steps into adulthood. At the end of a particularly lengthy and difficult military training that was conducted in heat so severe that two-thirds of my forty-person platoon became casualties to heatstroke, to celebrate our survival we held a talent show in the middle of nowhere. As the sun went down on the day and our time together, we paused to sing "America the Beautiful."

I love the true heart of humanity, and the most beautiful thing I have ever seen is the private sort of courage it takes to be willing to look at oneself with an open heart and an open mind, seeking only to know what is true.

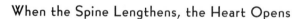

When the Spine Lengthens, the Heart Opens

Yoga offers us a natural progression to the practice of self-study that starts on the mat. We come to class and decide we like how we feel afterward. We like some of the teachers and we come to appreciate the dynamic community that has grown up around the practice. We learn new words and new perspectives. The workout on the mat starts to become a work-in. We begin noticing things like the way breathing slowly and deeply calms us down, and how we can sense the energy in the room. A mini life crisis occurs and we find that going to yoga helps. We are grateful to have yoga and feel a little sorry for those around us who do not. Our work-life starts to be informed by what we hear and experience in class. Some of the new friends we have made recommend books that they are finding helpful. As we reread a passage in one it feels like we are seeing something for the first time, something that was always there. On our mat a few days later the teacher suggests that we take our seat with a long, light spine, and when our spine lengthens we feel our heart opening.

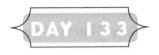

The Middle

My friend Matthew Sanford teaches the concept of noticing subtle sensation; he calls this "the middle." The start of the practice is entirely about the musculoskeletal system and paying attention to how muscle and bone stay upright and move against gravity. Then, one day, we start to notice how we are breathing and how we are feeling. We start to invest ourselves in the way we are being in a pose and what we are feeling while in it. This is the middle, when the mind has started to turn inward. Our perception of the body and the breath starts to change; how we feel starts to matter as much as what we think. We start to make decisions differently, pausing to notice how we feel about something before we act. From the middle we can see that we are not our thoughts, and that the space between our thoughts is a place we can rest in. If we are not our thoughts, then who are we? And who is resting in this new space I've found? This is the beginning of self-study.

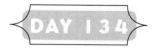

Learning from Others About Ourselves

The first context in which I made a concerted effort to become self-aware was a twelve-step community. Within that community there is the practice of reading teachings, but the primary tradition is an oral one, people passing on what they have learned to one another through the spoken word. Yoga is like that, teacher to student, student becoming teacher, teacher to student. I learned to learn by learning to listen. An oral tradition tends to exist within a sentence or two. Wisdom captured in the turn of a phrase. Here are a few of my favorites when it comes to self-study: How we see the problem is the problem. We see the world not as it is but as we are. Learn to reflect on the mind rather than to react from it. I didn't know that I didn't know. My way makes sense to me.

It seems likely that someone could develop an effective practice of self-study from the insights passed down within an oral tradition. But that was not the case for me. I needed the sort of intellectual framework that only books can provide. Not only that, I needed the words of the great teachers laid out comprehensively. I needed a map of the entire terrain in order to find my place and my way.

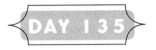

Wisdom Teachings

The first wisdom teachings I was exposed to were the writings of Bill Wilson, the founder of the twelve-step movement. From his books I was able to determine the true nature of my addiction and to understand its treatment. Bill Wilson experienced a spiritual awakening, and after reading his first book, I experienced one of my own. His teachings showed me what a rewarding life after alcohol might look like. In fact, the life I live today is largely thanks to his example. Bill Wilson inspired in me a lifelong passion for learning, which led me to the teachings of Lao-tzu and Deepak Chopra. From these teachers I learned the power of combining intention with non-attached involvement. They also made a poetic case for letting go with faith and taking delight in whatever the moment brings. The Buddha arrived on my radar at about the time I became a parent. The impact of the Buddha's teachings on my life is hard to capture in words. It's as if I was trapped in the story of my life and now I am living in the truth of it, the felt reality of it. And all of this learning, for which there are no words of gratitude big enough to suffice, appears to have been codified in the Yoga Sutras. A quarter of a century into the study of wisdom teachings I am of the belief that humanity has a magnificent grasp of its potential and a consensus on how to achieve it. The solution has been within reach for as long as we have been seeking it, but more often than not we are asking the wrong questions. This book is meant to help with that.

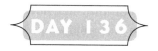

Insight

At the heart of wisdom teachings is our ability to arrive at genuine insight into the nature of reality and our relationship to it. I went around a room full of teachers and asked them each to share an insight they'd had that year, and all of them were able to with ease. Insight happens; it happens to us all the time, it is part of how we move through our lives, but it is not actively recognized and is rarely cultivated. We just know stuff, we just let go of stuff, we just understand something we never could before, a piece of the puzzle suddenly fits. Any successful creative endeavor features moments of genuine insight; a new direction, a new solution, a new way of being flows out of them. Lao-tzu wrote that the Tao is nowhere to be found yet it nourishes and completes all things. No creative work is complete without the nourishment of insight. Most moments of insight are ripples in ordinary consciousness, there for a moment, then gone. The curtain is pulled back an inch, then it falls back in place. What the person who caught the glimpse does with it is up to the individual. One of the reasons people choose to practice yoga is to follow up on what they glimpsed behind the curtain. A wisdom teaching like the Yoga Sutras is not a glimpse, it is the whole whack; the curtain is pulled back completely and someone has taken notes. The value of this kind of document grows in our lives as we do. We learn to know insight when we hear it, and each time we hear insight we get better at listening to it.

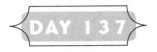

It's Important That I Teach Yoga

An example of an ordinary moment of insight in my life came during a phone call. I was being offered my first job as a yoga teacher, and during the phone call I suddenly knew it's important that I teach yoga. At the time of the call I was a social work graduate student and I had a tremendous amount of passion for the work I was doing. It was my calling, it was my path, it was where my heart was, it was my way of saying thank you to the higher power that had given me my life back. I had been open to teaching because I had been trained to teach, I loved yoga, and I needed a part-time job. I was not looking for another career.

Despite all that, I had had a moment of insight like this before. The moment I got sober something let me know it was going to be okay, and it was. This was the same sort of awareness. The word that came to me as I listened on the phone was "important." I felt that I was being told that it was important that I teach yoga with the odd clarity we experience during intense moments of déjà vu. We are both remembering and understanding at the same time. I continued my studies but began to take yoga teaching seriously, finding as many opportunities to teach as I could. Four years later I was writing *Meditations from the Mat*. Today I am still teaching yoga and I still don't know why this is my path—the insight didn't cover that—only that it is my path.

CHAPTER THREE

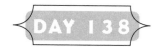

Not Knowing

The problem with insight is that it is as if each generation is supposed to build a puzzle and the puzzle pieces are scattered across the globe. These puzzle pieces are insights and callings, creative visions and heart songs, hatreds and wounds that will never heal. This one is a piece of the puzzle of beauty, this one courage, this one tragedy, this one vengeance, this one wisdom, this one forgiveness, this one the builder, this one the destroyer. Each of us knows our puzzle piece matters but we don't know how they all go together. The great teachers saw how. This is their gift, knowing how the puzzle is made up, what it should look like—what it will look like—what it looks like in the life we have already lived and are about to live. And when we hear them, we know they speak the truth. When we learn that Christ's last words included "Forgive them, for they know not what they do," and that the Buddha taught that we should "forgive everybody for everything," our hearts are stirred not only by the kindness but by the truth. The study of wisdom teachings gives us the courage and clarity to share our pieces of the puzzle with one another with wisdom and compassion.

DAY 139

Ali

In the house I grew up in sports was a religion. Our teachers were the women and men who had learned to excel in spite of it all, whose triumphs were honestly gained through blood, sweat, and tears. Of all the greats from that time, Muhammad Ali was ... well, he was the greatest. We loved him because he took boxing—something plain, something simple, something ugly—and made it beautiful. He took being African American—something beaten, something unspoken, something tragic—and made it triumphant. He took being himself and made it spectacular. He was a glimpse, for all who chose to see, of what it is to be a piece of the puzzle and share that piece with courage, joy, wisdom, and compassion.

DAY 140

The Map and the Compass

Our yoga practice equips us with a map in the form of wisdom teachings and a compass in the form of an open heart. There is a period of practice and study while we become available to the teachings and practices of yoga, then familiar with them. Our experience of the body, the breath, and the moment undergoes a profound shift. The teachings of yoga awaken our hearts and bring peace to our minds. We become ready to move from the middle toward freedom from what Bill Wilson and Albert Einstein described as "the bondage of self" and the "prison of [one's] own ideas," respectively.

Why the prep time? Why not just jump in? Did any of the saints from any period in history do handstands and alternate-nostril breathing? Maybe not, but saints happen fairly randomly. Yoga offers anyone the chance to become self-aware and eventually achieve what Lao-tzu termed "freedom from his own ideas." This seems worth the trouble. The practice works on every level of our being simultaneously. Through the embodied practices of asana, *pranayama*, and meditation we begin to heal the body and awaken the heart, and through the study of wisdom teachings we begin to heal the mind and awaken the heart. Like the chakras, our practice comes together at the heart. It meets in the middle. And from the middle we can begin to reflect on the mind rather than react from it.

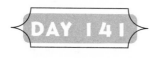

Getting Out of Our Own Way

The simplest explanation for why we should bother with self-study is that we all know the experience of needing to get out of our own way. We can be leaders, followers, moms, dads, yoga students, yoga teachers, tinkers, tailors, soldiers, or spies. Whatever hat we choose to put on, we still get in our own way. We can be right or wrong, having our worst day or our best, and there we are, standing between ourselves and the moment we find ourselves in. On my wedding day I spent much of the time making sure other people were happy, rather than focusing on the wonder of the moment. Without a map and compass to get us there we seem destined to live a block or two from the actual experience of life.

The compass and the map confirm what clinical research has begun to discover and yoga has known for several millennia, that we share three primary survival strategies with all living beings: creating separations; maintaining stability; approaching opportunities and avoiding threats. These strategies work great for survival, but for the human that possesses world-class pattern-recognition abilities, the fact that our survival strategies are temporary at best, doomed to fail at worst just doesn't sit well. The life we have and the life we want are rarely one and the same. What the compass and the map reveal is that things don't need to change—we do.

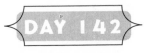

Creating Separations

Creating separations is the survival strategy that lets us know it's important to tell our children which berries to eat and which berries to avoid. But it doesn't stop there; it feels like the world needs to conform to our preferences. "Keep off my grass!" "No people like that in our church or in our schools!" "No one in my spot at the yoga studio!" Our efforts to create separations and clear distinctions between "yours" and "mine" have been almost as inventive as reality has been at undermining them. Separations just don't last in a universe in which everything is connected. The Buddha taught that our practice of self-study can begin with noticing, just noticing, when we want and when we don't want. We have learned to be right there at the beginning of the in-breath, and now we are being asked to be right there in the midst of wanting and not wanting, right there, not judging, not wishing, just seeking to know what is true here, now.

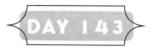

Nonattached Involvement

Paying a little bit of attention in the midst of wanting and not wanting reveals a self that is opposed to the way things are, not just right now but fundamentally. If I get my ducks in a row they should stay that way. Burnout, stress, anger, addiction, and narcissism don't seem to help; even lawyers, guns, and money won't make those ducks stay in line.

So we refer to the map that wisdom teachings give us and remind ourselves that we can take an action while letting go of the result, that we can just be right there in the action itself. As we refer to the compass of our hearts, we know that being right there will work, that being right there was the point all along.

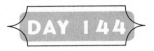

Maintaining Stability

A friend of mine recommended an accountant he claimed had saved him a lot of money. Two years later, as I was going through the litigious dissolution of a business partnership, the Internal Revenue Service audited my personal taxes and asked me to pay them an additional sixty thousand dollars. In the course of that year I was forced to sell the house I grew up in and went several hundred thousand dollars into debt. With my wife pregnant with our second child, I moved my family out of state for work.

There have been only a handful of moments in my fifty years of life that equaled the suffering I experienced during this time. The humbling experience of this series of setbacks and losses has played a critical and positive role in the well-being I now experience in my life. It was a very loud call to practice self-study. It woke me up from the slumber my "success" had visited on me. Upon awakening, I saw the beauty of the life I lived and that it was made up of people who were giving me more than they were receiving. As odd as it sounds, teaching yoga had pulled me away from practicing yoga. I had spent the last five years prioritizing my professional life over my personal life, and that is just a very bad trade. I could be counted on in the classroom but not really anywhere else. Without the pain of seeing how I had become less of a friend, less of a husband, less of a father, as I became more of a "success," the next level of my yoga practice would never have happened. My friend Todd Norian says that when things are difficult you are about to get a promotion. Eckhart Tolle wrote that when the fabric of our life is torn, God shines through. Maintaining stability in your life is good, but sometimes life has something even better in mind.

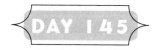

The Fabric of Our Life

I believe that sometimes hard times come to us to let us know that the life we are trying to maintain has been cut from the wrong cloth. This has certainly been the case for me, and in the years since my own difficulties I have coached and been a teacher to hundreds of people going through difficult chapters in their lives. With the exception of the loss of a loved one, what they were losing was a life they had outgrown. What they were learning is that the fabric of our life is in a constant state of flux. The child thinks her world is built out of stone. The adult learns that our lives are built from sand blown by the wind, forming one moment, then dissolving and re-forming the next. The smile of an adult is the smile of one who has learned to love each fleeting experience and knows that the wind that will sweep away this cherished moment is the same wind that will sweep in the next.

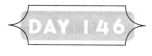

Flow

In yoga, rather than finding stability we discover balance and flow. When we consult the map of our wisdom teachings, it tells us that we have thought the impermanent was permanent, and that our resulting efforts to live backward have caused us to suffer. When we consult the compass of our hearts

CHAPTER THREE

we know this to be true. We find ourselves ready to ask the right question: "If my world is in constant flux, what does stability look like?" The answer we receive from our practice is flow—the ability to act and to let go at the same time. Planning a day with children is a great way to practice flow. The plan creates an outline and gets the family out the door. It might even point you in the right direction, but at some point we can cling to our plan and suffer or we can let go and flow with the joy of being a family on an adventure. Happy parents have learned to flow. If we fight against the waves they will beat us relentlessly, but if we flow with them they will take us on the ride of a lifetime.

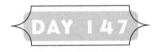

An Appropriate Response

My teachers tell me that the Buddha described enlightenment as "an appropriate response." I have greeted this teaching with a mixture of appreciation and disappointment depending on whether my glass is half-full or half-empty. When it is half-empty, I feel as though something more substantial than "an appropriate response" would not be too much to ask for. When I am a little more on my game, I am heartened by the fact that none other than the Buddha himself recognized what my life comes down to. I cannot fix anything forever, or learn anything forever, or maintain anything forever; I can only respond, appropriately, to whatever the moment brings. An appropriate response is a momentary blending of energies: a little patience, a little decisiveness, a little listening, a little asking, some walking away, and about the same amount of walking toward. Each yoga pose expresses discipline and freedom, steadiness, and ease. Each breath is a full measure of emptiness balanced by an equal measure of fullness. In meditation the heart and mind become empty to take in the moment fully. The practices we use to develop our ability to have an appropriate response are themselves an appropriate response.

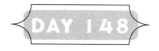

Approaching Opportunities

When we are children opportunities tend to be singular events, like Christmas and a trip to the candy store. They come and they go. Before is great, during is even better, and after is no fun at all. Each event is a discrete moment that breaks the general pattern of our young lives. As an adult, things tend to pile up: waiting for this opportunity for years while negotiating the reality of two or three others and mourning the loss of yet another. Whether we are willing to admit it or not, we often have more opportunities than we can adequately address while craving the next opportunity. The Yoga Sutras tell us that our skewed relationship to opportunity reflects our skewed relationship to ourselves and our world.

In our confusion we cannot see each opportunity for what it is. Some will be great, then fade; some will never come; some will be fantastic but stay way too long; and none will be a replacement for the felt sense of this body, this breath, this moment, this calmly abiding heart, this spacious awareness. Calmly established in the present moment, opportunities are like the weather, a unique blend of energies to be experienced fully, met in the same way as Rob Machado meets the next section of his eternal wave in

Indo. The wave and the surfer complete a moment together, each offering the other a second or two of self-definition but no more. We see the size and shape of the wave because of the scale the surfer gives it. We see the courage and ability of the surfer because of the size and shape of the wave. That is all an opportunity will ever be—a wave well surfed.

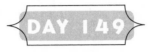

Avoiding the Unpleasant

The Yoga Sutras tell us that "future suffering can be avoided," and I would add that while this is true, it is also true that doing so is pretty much a full-time job. For the proactive among us this is really good news. Yoga is not a fatalistic practice of numbed-out resignation. It is a proactive one, in which we study the habits that cause us to suffer and establish skillful habits in their stead.

Paradoxically, one of the habits that cause us to suffer is the habit of avoiding the unpleasant. Our attempts at avoiding, or at least managing, necessary pain, for example, pose a challenge in every area of our life from fitness to nutrition to personal growth. Most folks, when they sit to meditate, find it uncomfortable, difficult, and boring all at the same time, and quit. The equation seems to be that if something is uncomfortable we should avoid it no matter what. Swami Vivekananda suggested that we quit nibbling at things; I would suggest we stop tap-dancing around them. Brené Brown teaches us to lean into the discomfort. That is a great place to start: keep it simple and start on your mat and your cushion, staying right there as you hold the pose a little longer.

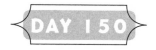

Whatever the Moment Brings

After breakfast my children clean their rooms and I clean the kitchen. When each of us is done, we meet in the living room and clean it together. My children are of an age where they like to be given small tasks that they can do on their own and take pride in. They like the way their room feels when everything is put away and they find a deep contentment with the space life has provided for them. We all tend to meet the task with more than enough energy to be successful because of the meal we have just eaten and because we are together. Each time we clean we discover things about our home and ourselves that we had forgotten and that we are happy to be able to share with one another. This week my daughter, Jasmine, found a toy monkey that our dog, Chelsea, had treated very roughly when she was a puppy. Jasmine bandaged the monkey quite skillfully and we reflected on how much both Chelsea and my daughter had changed, and how they were still very much the same. Met in this fashion, the necessity of keeping the house clean becomes an opportunity to come together and enjoy one another while getting better at life. Purity, contentment, zeal, and self-study turn our practice into a self-sustaining way of life, a set of choices with which to meet any moment.

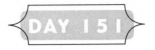

Isvara-pranidhana

Consider the power of the choices we have made up till now. The practice of the *yamas* not only prevents us from squandering our energy in negative patterns, it provides us with a set of practices that generate more energy than we put into them. Ask anyone how much energy they put into a true act of kindness (the codependent kind doesn't have the same effect) and they will not be able to remember; all they will remember is how glad they are for having had the opportunity and how good they felt afterward. While the *yamas* concern the choices we are making in the world, the *niyamas* bring that same skill into our relationship with our self. Purity, contentment, zeal, and self-study practiced consistently create the possibility of an ever-increasing happiness and freedom. The final *niyama*, *isvara-pranidhana* ("surrender to God"), closes the loop, directing all this positive energy, all this life, toward the realization of our core values and beliefs.

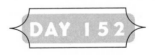

Right There

The essence of yoga is captured in learning to be right there at the beginning of the in-breath, learning to aim our attention and feel into the quality of our connection or disconnection with our own felt experience. This idea of aiming our attention seems like a minor detail until you consider the level of disconnect humanity is presently struggling with.

We seem to think that saying there is alignment between our actions and our values is enough. That saying it or thinking it makes it so. I believe this is what suffering helps me with. It's just life's feedback. It's life's way of drawing my attention right there to the gap between who I think I am and what I think I am doing, and reality. Yoga is offering us a way to be right there, without the suffering and turmoil, by first teaching us how to pay attention.

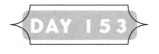

Something Greater

You hit what you aim at.

Zig Ziglar

The first line of the Yoga Sutras is "And now the practice of yoga." It assumes that we have been out doing our research looking for love in all the wrong places and provides us with a reality rehab. It starts by aiming our attention at something close by and easy to hit, like our hands and feet, and progresses to something a little subtler, like the rise and fall of our breathing. Eventually we get around to placing our attention on how things feel and the way we think about them. Watching the movements of our thoughts brings our attention to the space between them the way watching shadows pass across the surface of the ocean brings our attention to the ocean. The shadows are moving, so our eye catches them first, but in time it is the ocean that captures our imagination. We begin to connect to the larger part of ourselves and to aim our attention there. Whatever our original motivation had been in coming to yoga is eventually abandoned as we begin to aim our practice and our lives at something greater.

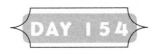

Alignment

I teach that yoga is the alignment of our values and our actions through the application of its principles and practices, and that the relevance of yoga in anyone's life is found in its ability to serve that function. Much of yoga can be found right there in the everyday work of putting our beliefs into practice, and for many years after we begin practicing, yoga is a pragmatic process of putting out the fires we have set for ourselves and the slow accumulation of behaviors that yield more energy than we put into them, like kindness and generosity. Eventually, though, we must take responsibility for the big questions. What am I aiming my life at and why? If I am clear about how I wish to live my life, am I aligned behind that life or am I still living in the shadows of one I've outgrown? Am I dedicating my life to something, or am I making things up as I go along? This is the work of *isvara-pranidhana*.

A few years ago, a lot of people were wearing bracelets that asked, "What would Jesus do?" It's a great question. In Buddhism you learn to find support from the Buddha's example. It helps to pause and reflect on the fact that you are taking your seat to meditate just as the Buddha took his seat and to take refuge in the fact of his ultimate victory. Effective spiritual practice is aimed at an ideal, and in my experience that ideal, however lofty, is realizable by anyone who practices sincerely. It's as if the ideal becomes a prayer or a vision for the person holding it and her footsteps unerringly find their way to it.

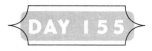

Role Models

For some, avatars like Jesus and the Buddha are perfect ideals to aim their life toward. They see the qualities they seek in their own lives demonstrated in the lives of these great teachers. For me, that has always been too abstract a connection. My ideal has been made out of the lives of ordinary women and men. I am inspired by the heart-stopping manner in which each of us has the potential to turn an ordinary moment into an extra-ordinary one, an ordinary action into something of lasting beauty. I am inspired by moments in people's lives and by skills and habits that play out over their entire lifetimes. I consider whatever success I meet with on a given day due in part to the way others have taught me how to live by their example.

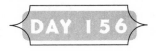

Equanimity

Both of my children had Beth Landry as their kindergarten teacher. As their parent, there are no words to describe the gratitude I feel when I reflect on this. She is kindness and wisdom with a smile, and my children learned what school was from her. The classroom she presides over contains a throng of five-year-olds, and she guides their day like the conductor of an orchestra. After the children leave at 1:20 she works until five to get the classroom ready for the next day. She keeps this pace going ten months a year and has done so for the last thirty-two years with no sign of slowing down. I have known her now for seven years and I have never seen her complain or waver. She believes in what she does and does it with a smile. This is the equanimity with which I would like to carry out my responsibilities to myself, to my family, and to my community.

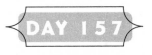

Heart

Kelly Slater won his first world title when he was twenty years old and went on to win five more before retiring from surfing at the height of his powers. Three years later he returned to surfing and would battle for another four years before earning his seventh world title. He is now in his forties and still one of the world's top competitive surfers, having won an unheard-of eleven titles. His extraordinary success is often thought of as his defining characteristic. For me, though, it is how he handled life without success that matters the most. Between his sixth and seventh world titles there were seven long, uncertain years in which he never stopped working on himself and his surfing. For seven long years he never stopped believing in himself and in his art. This is how I want to work and believe as a husband, a father, a teacher, a human being.

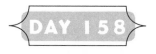

Courage

My older sister, Wendy, was the first one of my siblings to do anything. She was the first to go to middle school, the first to go high school, the first to leave home for college. These days it is my daughter Jasmine's turn to be first. In both cases I have been in awe of the eldest child's place in things, to step out into the complete unknown at each stage of your life. My most cherished pictures are of Jasmine from her first day at pre-K and her first day in kindergarten. There is a smile on her face and the light of high adventure in her eyes. She goes with the hearts of her family and she has no doubt that she will make us proud. This is the courage with which I want to step out into the unknown, the courage of the eldest child.

Rest in peace, Wendy; it was an honor to be your brother and it is an honor to carry your memory.

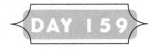

THE SPIRIT OF PRACTICE

Kindness

My wife, Mariam, is the eldest of five and cared for each of her younger siblings while she was growing up. All the memories she has shared with me about her childhood have to do with caretaking; there are no stories of playing games or going shopping, just looking after her brothers and sisters, wanting the best for them. Once she became a mom it was a thing to see. When our children were very young she did not blink at the work it took to care for them. Day after day, year after year, she withstood the constant, grueling, messy work of raising kids without so much as a glance for the exit. As our children have grown older, she has kept track of a never-ending list of details to make sure they are on time with the right homework assignment, sports equipment, birthday present, field trip permission slip, or extra-special snack to take the edge off testing week. She does their homework with them and follows up with their teachers. She sweats all of the details, from soccer sign-ups, to theater camp, to playdates, to the type of lock our daughter will need to be familiar with when she starts middle school in the fall. Mariam loves the people in her life every second of every day. This is how I want to love.

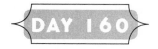

Answering the Call of Duty

A moment that inspires me whenever I think of it is the last moment of the life of a woman whose name I will never know and whose cause I have no sympathy for.

She is remembered as "the blond woman," and she fought at Gettysburg on the Confederate side. There was a tradition in some regiments that if someone died, a family member could take their place. In this case it was a wife who took her husband's position in a Virginia regiment. She charged with General Pickett's division on the last horrific day of that fateful battle. They crossed a mile of open ground, uphill and under heavy fire from three sides. Some of them made it to the top of the hill; a few of them made it to a stone wall that is said to have been the farthest point of the Confederate advance. She died there, amidst her comrades, a pistol in each hand, both barrels empty. The beauty that I love deserves no less from me.

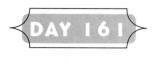

Surrender

The final skill of the *niyamas* is the ability to surrender yourself to the life you have chosen. I am preparing myself for a photo shoot, images of which will be in this book. I am content to work with the time that I have, the body that I have, and the coaching that I have. I am self-aware and know that nutrition, what I eat, will make up 80 percent of my preparation. My coach has given me a food plan that is both intellectually sound and has made me feel good when I am on it. The role models who inspire me the most have modeled a willingness to do the kind of work I am doing now with nutrition. I am working with a coach because I know that intensity and commitment come easier when you are on a team. All that is left for me to be successful is to surrender to the choice that I have made, one day at a time.

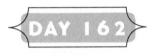

Grace

As a part of my training as a military officer, I went to the U.S. Army Airborne School at Fort Benning, Georgia. I took a three-week course, culminating in a "Jump Week," in which you jump out of various types of military aircraft. Upon completion of five jumps you get your Airborne wings, the memory of which still brings a smile to my face. In the first week a lot of attention is given to how you stand in the door of the aircraft before jumping out. There is even instruction on how you are supposed to check the exterior of the aircraft before jumping. Many of us would later comment that this training must have been for jumping out of a slowly moving truck, because at 180 miles per hour it was completely unnecessary. If you are willing to jump out of an airplane you simply need to walk toward the door. At some point well before you actually get to the door you get swept up. Grace is like that. If you are willing to aim your life at an ideal you simply need to walk toward it. At some point, grace will sweep you up.

THREE WAYS TO EMBRACE THE SPIRIT OF PRACTICE

Make lists of:

1) The virtues you wish to express with your practice
2) The virtues you wish to express with your life
3) The role models who have embodied those virtues for you

Reflect on these lists often.

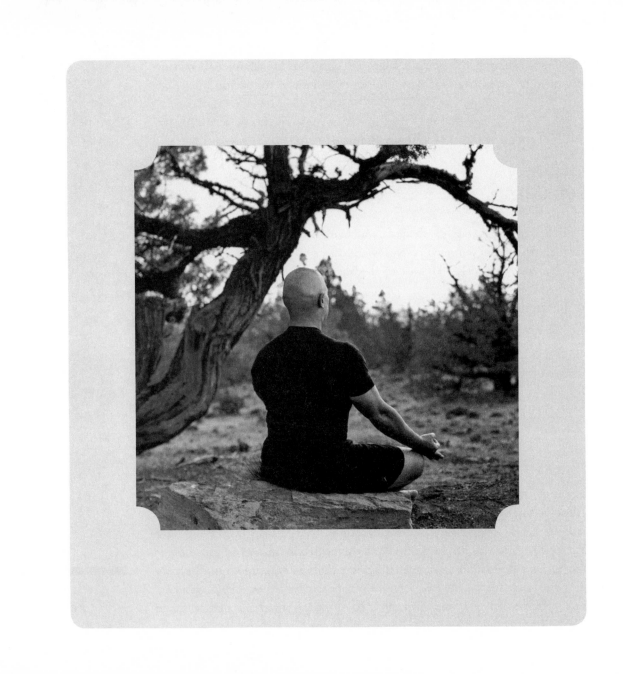

CHAPTER FOUR

MINDFULNESS

> *When you change the way you see the world,*
> *the world you see changes.*

Wayne Dyer

Mindfulness is the ability to see things as they are, free from the filter of our conditioning. It is this crucial capacity that creates the space in which loving-kindness and compassion are possible. The cultivation of mindfulness allows us to break free from the multidimensional influences of our time and our place in the world—our family history, our cultural biases, our personal and professional experiences—and to begin to see what is true about ourselves and our world.

The first chapter of the Yoga Sutras lays out how to see, what to see, and how to relate to what you are seeing. In this first chapter, the student of yoga is taught to cultivate two abilities that, when combined, will allow her to see things as they are. They are *abhyasa*, the will to align and repeatedly realign our attention with the present moment, and *vairagya*, the ability to allow an experience to arise and pass without reacting to it.

The first discipline of yogic mindfulness is the ability to align with the present moment (*abhyasa*). Six of yoga's eight limbs train the individual to do just that. We begin with the poses. In the style of yoga asana I teach, we practice one pose after the next for ninety minutes, stretching the new student's ability to pay attention. Over time the experienced asana practitioner either gets used to practicing yoga with a distracted mind or begins to cultivate true powers of concentration, taking each moment, each breath, and each pose as it comes without leaning into the next moment.

The next capacity she develops is the ability to take each pose as it comes without reacting to it, learning to see and be without commentary (*vairagya*). She discovers within herself the ability to enjoy "dropping in" to an experience, allowing it to unfold in its own time and relating to it directly through her own felt experience. This maturation process in the student of

CHAPTER FOUR

153

asana is a profound transformation. Often without knowing it the student has prepared herself for the disciplines of yoga.

Mindfulness is also a healing practice in its own right. The degree to which humanity suffers from a disturbed mind cannot be overstated. The suffering that can be seen on any given day in any given place on the faces of the people who share our world as they contend with an inner life that is literally out of control is tragic. It is commonplace for people to hurt themselves or others in an attempt to resolve the seemingly endless suffering they are experiencing within the dream world of their own mind. Mindfulness effectively ends this suffering.

With *abhyasa* and *vairagya* we are able to reflect on the mind as opposed to reacting to it. Over time we are able to see our mental habits for what they are, just old programming whose aim was justified at one point in our life but may not be relevant today. Many of the assumptions I was born into fifty years ago are no longer congruent with the world I live in today. Reflecting on the mind as opposed to reacting to it, I am able to observe this and act accordingly. The practices of *abhyasa* and *vairagya* not only offer us this reflective ability, they teach us how to allow the mind to settle.

It is my experience that the mind is like a glass of water. If you set it down the water will return to its true nature, which is still and clear. Likewise the mind, left to its own devices, will settle and become awake, clear, and spacious. All that is needed for my mind to express its true nature is for me to allow it to. When the mind has returned to its original nature, so too does everything else, and the suffering we have come to associate with mental agitation ends.

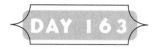

Effortlessness

In the past, people who embraced yoga would separate themselves from their culture, living apart from the everyday concerns of their peers. Whether they lived in monasteries or individual hermitages, these practitioners practiced, to the best of their ability, away from the influence of the world around them. In the U.S. these circumstances have been reversed. The adoption of yoga by the mainstream started with, and continues to be led by, the mainstream layperson in large cities and in small towns, the suburbs, the exurbs, and beyond. Who is practicing yoga has had a lot of influence on what yoga is today. It is dynamic, entrepreneurial, trendy, intelligent, playful, friendly, doing enormous good, and driven. This past week I had a conversation with a studio owner who shared with me her concerns over how manic yoga had become in Dallas. A few days later, I had the same conversation with a teacher from Boulder. While I understand their concern, I tend to take the long view. You have to start somewhere, and if trying to get a runner's high, or Madonna arms, from yoga gets you through the door, so be it. I believe even an overly vigorous asana practice raises a student's sensitivity and that she will eventually start making better choices for herself.

I started this book with a chapter on effortlessness because I do not believe you can learn about balance in a state of imbalance. Individually and collectively we are in a state of imbalance when it comes to over-efforting because we are still living from the logic of fear. Effortlessness is the inquiry into what we would do if we were not afraid. It asks, "How much and what kind of effort do we need to exert to be here now?"

CHAPTER FOUR

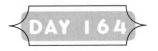

Nonviolence

For thousands of years people have studied the matter and they keep coming back to the same conclusion: violence makes things worse. The enormous physical harm that human violence causes each day creates a legacy of negative mental and emotional states that predisposes us to further violence. A teacher of mine put it simply: "Zen is not making things worse." Violence is not Zen. Violence of thought, violence of speech, violence of action, violence by omission, and influencing others to do violence makes our lives worse. The *yamas* help us to place our attention right there at the moment when we can choose violence or we can choose love.

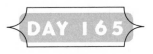

The Spirit of Practice

I teach teachers to bring a treat to each class. The treat is a special song, sequence of poses, way to teach a pose, or reading, something the teacher is excited to share with her students. This changes the energy of her relationship to the class. It is no longer something she has to do but rather something she is looking forward to doing. For most teachers, the first ten years are a long and winding learning curve featuring a lot of ups and downs, and the treat takes the edge off the downs. As she reflects on a less-than-great class, the teacher can at least feel good about the treat she shared. As she worries about the next class, she can focus on her excitement about sharing something new.

The *niyamas* do the same thing for our practice of yoga over the years. They are both an energetic foundation and a form of maintenance we can employ when things get stale. When I am in conflict or suffering around a situation, I do a quick inventory of the *yamas* to find how I am out of alignment. It always works. The same is true of the *niyamas*. If my practice has lost steam, there will be a *niyama* that can turn the lights back on.

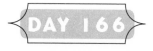

A Mind-made Prison

For most of us, the fact that we are living in what Einstein described as a mind-made prison of separateness becomes abundantly clear when we first begin to meditate. Our mind feels like a kind of echo chamber in which all we know and all we can experience is a repetitive stream of our own thoughts. The habit of thinking is so entrenched that it feels like the only process available to us. Yoga suggests there is another form of mental activity that we are well practiced in, only we do not think of it as an alternative to the suffering created by an overactive mind. To feel the temperature of a child's bath, to hear the wind rustle the leaves of a tree, to taste a spoonful of ice cream, we must shift our attention from thinking to feeling, or listening, or tasting. This shift provides us with a moment of pure awareness, with a moment of direct connection with what is *true here now*. It is normal and necessary for us to know what is true without the process of labeling or

CHAPTER FOUR

conceptualization, without creating a mind-made world or a mind-made self. Meditation empowers us to step out of our mind-made prison by recognizing a simple shift in the placement of our attention. It allows us to set ourselves free by coming to our senses.

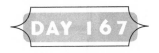

Nirodha

"*Nirodha*" is a Sanskrit word meaning "cessation." In Buddhism, suffering ceases. Within the twelve-step movement, the desire to use drugs or alcohol is lifted; it ceases. In yoga, the movements of the mind cease. In the systems I have studied and lived by there is an end to human suffering. *Nirodha* is not to be used as a measure of our present circumstances; rather it is meant to light our way.

Mindfulness is the ability to be present without opinion or commentary, and the ability to understand. I encourage you to bring mindfulness to your own experience of *nirodha*, both as part of the bigger picture—in the way that forms of suffering you have experienced in the past are no more—and in the ordinary moments that make up your day. Notice how, whenever you pause and take a breath, there it is, a moment of spacious peace; this is *nirodha*. Notice as you give yourself with ease and appreciation to the ordinary tasks that make up your day how there is the experience of timeless flow; this too is *nirodha*. Notice how each time you choose to withdraw your attention from a disturbing train of thought and breathe your way back into the vibrant present, the suffering you had a moment before has vanished. *Nirodha* is the ever-present truth hidden beneath the turbulence we create with our minds, the possibility that our suffering can end now.

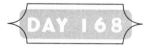

Bhavantu

A dear friend died this summer. She could see the room where her body was lying and her sister crying. She said that while she was dead she experienced complete peace and safety. But she also had a strong sense that her work in this lifetime was not done. She came back and is on the mend, but the experience of peace and safety has not left her. I have not died, but I have had a glimpse of the ground of our being, the ground of our existence, the manner in which we are held by the divine, and it was much the same as my friend's. To be touched by this understanding is to live each day with the desire that your life bears witness to the divine's love for us, to try in some way to convey what is beyond words. There is a simple Sanskrit word that captures both the knowing my friend experienced and the desire to share this knowing: "*bhavantu*." *Bhav* is the state of unification with the divine—what my friend experienced in death, what we experience in *nirodha*. *Antu* is the affirmation "May it be so, it must be so." May it be so.

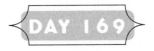

The Habits of the Mind

One of the challenges Westerners face when taking their yoga practice off the mat and onto their meditation cushion is a mistaken belief that meditation is about trying to stop the mind. In my experience the opposite is true. It was only after my meditation practice matured that I was able to use my mind at all. Before that I was not using my mind; I was reacting from habit and confusing habit with choice.

The mind is clear, spacious consciousness, like the water in a glass that has been still for a while. This clear, open space processes the input from both our outer and inner worlds, translating raw data into manageable concepts. It is not subject to inclinations like aversion and desire, in the same way that our hearing is without preference—it just hears; our mind just sees and, when asked to, creates meaning. It is not in the business of causing us to suffer. Where things get challenging is in the shorthand we have created to make the mind's job easier. Things get divided into packages of meaning. *This smell is good, that person is bad, I am good at math.* The highly nuanced and ever-changing nature of reality gets lost in the desire for efficiency. These chunks of meaning and the reactions they engender can be considered the habits of the mind. Our first experiences of watching the mind in meditation amount to the process of watching the habits of the mind at work busily offering yesterday's meaning to today's unprecedented events and going through its loops of hope and fear. This is so ingrained that we are unable to imagine the mind's true nature, or that our experience of it could be indescribably soothing. The practice of mindfulness begins by sorting out the difference between the habits of the mind and the mind itself, just as later we begin the practice of compassion by learning the difference between a person and a behavior.

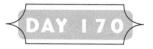

Noticing Nothing

The habits of the mind are so swift and effective at creating meaning that we often mistake the false world they concoct for reality. We do not say, "This is what I am seeing," or "This is the meaning I am making"; we say, "This is what is true and real. I was there. I saw it." Usually something truly drastic has to happen for us to question the way we habitually make meaning. Even then, it is still rare that we become fully aware of the ways that we are processing reality and begin to influence that processing through conscious intent (I hope this book will improve your odds). Those of us who have made it onto our meditation cushion have that opportunity. We begin by watching the body and the breath and eventually progress to watching our thoughts and feelings. With some time and effort we find ourselves able to watch the mind, first on our cushion and then in everyday life.

Like everything else, the mind is still and it moves. In stillness it is like a quiet pond. Then it moves to make meaning. This movement is like the ripples on the surface of the pond when a stone is thrown in. I began to have a healthy relationship with my mind when I began to notice what my mind felt like in the absence of ripples. What the mind is like when it is moving and what it is like when it is not. I began to notice *nirodha*, the calm, luminous nature of the mind when it ceases to move.

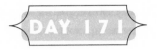

Nothing Special

We start out thinking the peace that yoga has to offer is special and only found after years of arduous practice. It is and it isn't. I have found far more peace than I thought was possible by applying the principles and practices of yoga consistently over the course of decades, but that peace was always there. It is there in the moments we take for granted, when the mind is still and the heart is open: cleaning our room, mowing the lawn, walking the dog, listening to a dear friend. Peace is most often found when we are doing nothing special. It's just that we don't recognize it for what it is and for what it demonstrates about the human condition. We think peace is found in the extraordinary—and it can be, only because it is already there in the ordinary. The extra-ordinary, the peak moments, just bring a sharpened focus to what was there when we were doing nothing special.

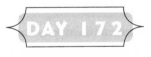

Asana

"Asana" is the Sanskrit word for "pose," and it begins the training of the mind in yoga. Asana, *pranayama* ("mindful breathing"), and meditation create the felt space within which the practice of mindfulness takes place. Asana trains the mind to be present for the felt experience of the body in an unambiguous fashion. We are either feeling into our feet or we are not. We are either balancing effort with ease in a pose or we are not. The inner rotation of the arms in downward dog is either balanced by the action of outer rotation or it is not. The body in a yoga pose is the perfect place to start learning how to aim and sustain our attention. The large life-resembling actions of asana grab the new student's attention in a way that the subtle shifts of attention in meditation often cannot. Moving through a series of poses, the student is immersed in sensation. When the mind is moving and when it is still becomes writ large. She starts to notice that if the mind moves it becomes hard to stay with the pose. When the mind is still the pose becomes something beautiful and alive. The student begins to realize she has a choice. Suffering isn't random; it's actually just a question of where she is placing her attention. The implications of this may not become clear all at once, but yoga never asks us to learn anything but by degrees.

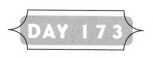

What Happens to the Mind When It's Listening to the Body

Meditation is not a singular act, something that you either do or do not do. Rather, it's a set of actions practiced until they become habits that net out to a new relationship with our mind. This is a worthy goal, but many people think it is unattainable. It's one of the reasons I love teaching asana, because it is such an easy way to get people past their belief that they cannot meditate. I start off with meditation on the body. In child pose, at the beginning of class, I ask my students to move from thinking to feeling. Then I include the breath. In downward dog, I have them focus on the fact that

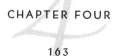

CHAPTER FOUR

they are breathing in when they are breathing in and that they are breathing out when they are breathing out. Then I include the energy body. In warrior two, I ask them to draw energy in and shine energy out . . . effortlessly. Then I include *nirodha*. In mountain pose, at the end of a vigorous sequence, I ask them to be in their feet in a way that allows them to lift and open their hearts, effortlessly, noticing what happens to the mind when it's listening to the body, and noticing what happens to the body when the mind is listening.

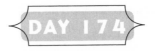

Evolving on Purpose

Mindfulness became absolutely essential in my life when my daughter was born. For the thirty-nine years leading up to her birth, being set in my ways had consequences, but these had always seemed manageable. The people for whom my way of doing things did not work could leave. With the birth of my daughter, Jasmine, it became apparent that I was now in a situation in which at least two people were stuck with me. If I was going to make our relationship work, I would have to be able to adjust my attitudes, actions, and reactions in real time. This was unprecedented. I was now in a situation in which my primary contribution was my ability to be present and make choices based not on my preferences or my conditioning but on my principles.

The stress of being a dinosaur in my own life caused me to seek out stillness, calm, and safety. I needed grounding badly. Meditation provided that, and in an instance of outrageous good fortune, it also provided me with the ability to change my mind as rapidly as my life was changing. When it became necessary, I discovered that I could evolve on purpose.

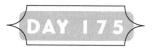

Halfway There

When I began attending silent meditation retreats, I learned something about my asana and *pranayama* practice. I discovered that they amounted to enormously effective meditation training. The challenge was to translate what I knew from those practices into a practice that featured holding the same pose for forty-five minutes . . . ten times a day. Eventually I would embrace walking meditation, but in the beginning it was all about the forty-five-minute seated posture. My mind went off. It was just too much to manage. I could think about something for twenty minutes or so, then fight against the discomfort for ten minutes or so, but at some point within a forty-five-minute pose I would run out of ways to manage, numb, or avoid my experience. To make matters worse the poses just kept coming. They wore me down. My ability to coerce or abandon what was coming up for me—my boredom, my fear, my resentment, my discomfort, my vulnerability, my being alive in this moment—just could not hold up under this pressure. I tried again and again to avoid suffering with the habits my mind had built up over a lifetime and the results just kept coming up short. This was unmanageable. Exhausted and defeated, I stopped managing and started breathing, feeling, and appreciating.

The habits of my mind were of no use to me, but the skills I had learned on my mat were. I found I could shift out of a mind running through its

CHAPTER FOUR

165

patterns, in hopes of escape, into a body that was both still and vibrant and a breath that was a calm breeze moving across a forest hillside. Instead of a way to manage reality or to avoid it entirely I discovered a way to be with life that was not only doable but felt like coming home. Once I surrendered I discovered that I was already halfway there.

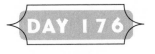

Abhyasa

Moving from thinking to feeling on my meditation cushion made a big difference in my practice and in my life. Through my body I was able to access the beauty of just being somewhere. First it was a bench at the retreat center, but eventually it became anywhere. These days I will stop what I am doing and just sit in my living room and do nothing but appreciate being in my living room. If I am talking to someone, I practice just appreciating being with that person, having that moment. On a plane, on a surfboard, at the end of the day sitting in a chair as my children brush their teeth and select the books they want to read, walking with my dog through the redwoods by my house, anywhere, anytime, is a good place, and a good time, to stop and appreciate life. Asana and *pranayama*—the postures and the mindful breathing of yoga—equip you for this practice.

What my early meditation retreats forced upon me was the ability to appreciate life regularly. To survive a series of forty-five-minute postures you have to move out of your head and into the moment. I had learned a new reaction to being somewhere. Instead of immediately moving into the intellectual process of how my circumstance *relates to me*, I was learning to move into the felt process of *relating to that circumstance. Abhyasa*, or "practice," is the logical next step in learning to appreciate being in a place. It is the practice of repeatedly aligning and realigning the mind to the present moment. *Abhyasa* is learning to be "right here" over and over again until it becomes a habit of the mind.

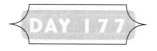

Collecting and Unifying the Mind

My teachers tend to treat the first few days of a meditation retreat as a time when nothing much is happening. They suggest we allow ourselves to take naps and deal with having just left our overcaffeinated, overstimulated daily existence. While we are napping and working on letting go of whatever trivialities we've been attached to, we are guided through the process of collecting and unifying the mind. My teachers are the kinds of people who attend six-month meditation retreats in the jungles of Thailand, so I can understand how underwhelmed they are by the "quality of practice" in the room on day two of a ten-day retreat in the privileged comfyness of Marin County, California. My experience of those first few days is very different from theirs. For me, ten days of practice anywhere is actually fairly hardcore and the early days have a big impact.

To help us to collect and unify our minds, the teachers give us a very simple instruction that we are to follow for three or four days in a row: to be right there at the beginning of the in-breath. That is all. Over and over again, to know that we are breathing when we are breathing, to practice *abhyasa*. Within a day or so I begin to notice a marked increase in the ambi-

CHAPTER FOUR

ent stillness of my mind. Shortly after that I find my mind inclined toward resting easily on the breath, or the way a lizard moves across a rock, or the taste of Earl Grey tea. Not only has my mind developed a powerful ability to focus, it has developed the radiant quality of *nirodha*, the "cessation" of my overly busy thoughts. The loops of distraction are still playing, but they are starting to be drowned out by the stillness of focus, the beauty a focused mind can perceive, and the vibrant spaciousness of the mind at rest. My dreams start to become extremely vivid because my mind is no longer exhausted at the end of the day. Collected and unified, it is starting to choose quality over quantity.

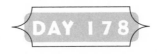

Momentum

The momentum of distraction is actually quite weak, like a small wheel that needs constant pushing to keep spinning. The momentum of the mind's ability to be powerfully focused is much greater, like a large stone wheel that's hard to get moving but once it starts spinning can keep going for ages. *Abhyasa* gets that stone wheel spinning. Within a couple of days of steady effort on retreat, you begin to explore this quality of the mind, how deeper levels of concentration have a self-sustaining quality. The mind shifts from its usual state of distraction and finds that it prefers to be awake. Each new object it takes up is explored in detail. Colors, smells, tastes, textures, and sounds take on a fascinating depth. My teachers are big into wearing thick socks and shawls, and after a few days you understand why—they are more sensitive to cold because they are more sensitive to everything. Having learned to establish this sort of concentration on retreat I have learned to be able to return to it in my home practice by setting aside just a couple of hours once or twice a week for a slightly deeper period of walking and sitting meditation, or asana and meditation. The sustained level of concentration my practice affords me has increased my effectiveness in every area of my life.

Once this type of concentration is learned we can begin to watch the mind in earnest.

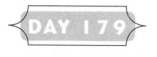

Contrast

Silence and sound define each other; one cannot be understood without the other. Watching the mind is much the same. We cannot understand the habits of the mind without first experiencing the luminous stillness of *nirodha*. Collecting and unifying the mind is a necessary first step toward understanding how it works. It serves the dual purpose of providing us with the ability to hold our attention steadily on something while also providing us with the felt experience of when our minds are not in distraction or contraction. With the mind in concentration, we experience emotional well-being and the ability to choose where to direct our attention. Once we have established our concentration, the habits of the mind are no longer experienced as reality, or normal, but rather are seen for what they are: artificial projections that are generated automatically based on external or internal stimuli. They are patterns that are based on at best accurate assessments of past circumstances and at worst misunderstandings inherited from our families and communities. In either case, the habits of our mind were formed in the past and their relevance to the present is yet to be determined. The practice of mindfulness allows us to choose what works and to let go of the rest.

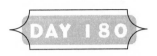

Achieving Lift-off

With the practice of *abhyasa*, we are beginning to pay attention on purpose. Whether we are on our mat, on our cushion, or listening to someone on the phone, we begin to notice when the mind wanders and to bring it back to the present moment. The physical practices of asana, *pranayama*, and meditation are teaching us to not only bring attention back to the moment but to embody it as well, returning to proper posture and proper breathing. A sign that you are back in the present is often a deep breath. For a while it is enough to know you are here now and to enjoy a long, slow breath in and out, feeling as though you have just awoken from a stressful dream and are glad to be back in your own life. Eventually you realize that the full breath is needed because of the effort it takes to leave the present moment and how the body has had to contract around that effort in order for you to stay gone.

This effort to achieve lift-off from the present moment is perceptible as a contraction of the body and a shortening of the breath. Asana and *pranayama* have taught us to be sensitive to just this sort of contraction and prepared us to soften back into our connection to the present. We are learning that it takes effort to leave the present and that it is effortless to return. Being here is easier.

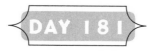

Contracted States

The fact that we have to contract around the effort to leave the present sheds a new light on the practices of asana and *pranayama* and explains the Zen teaching that "to take the right posture is to take the right frame of mind." When grounded in the body and the breath, the mind is in *nirodha* and the body is without the tension of what my teachers call the contracted states of wanting, not wanting, and delusion. Then the mind turns toward an external or internal stimulus, contracting into a habitual way of relating to the stimulus. *This should not be, this should be, I want this, I don't want that.* This mental contraction shows up in the body and the breath as well. The mind may treat this as business as usual but the body knows better as it experiences the contraction.

With practice, we come to recognize the connection between the contracted states and the experience of suffering. Sitting and breathing effortlessly, we notice that the mind has latched on to something, and with this grasping there is a contraction of the body and the breath. To realign with the present moment we can detach the mind from what it is grasping, but it is easier simply to move from thinking back to feeling, to use our training in *pranayama* and asana to bring the body into effortless uprightness and the breath into effortless fullness. As we get better at this in meditation, we begin to see it show up in our everyday lives. Caught in a contraction, we simply return to this body, this breath, this moment, and realize we have a choice when we did not know we had one.

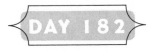
Leapfrog

Suffering is not a monolithic experience; rather, it is a semipermanent game of leapfrog, with the mind hopping from one contracted state to the next. *I want this to happen, I don't want that to happen, This should never have happened, I hope that will happen.* If we are not contracted around a specific outcome, like not being late for work, we contract around vague worries and hopes. What is termed "body image issues" these days is a protracted contraction around not wanting what is thought to be present, and wanting what is thought to be absent. We call the experience of these states "stress" and are attributing an ever-increasing list of illnesses to it. It makes sense to me. Using our minds, our hearts, and our bodies to hold on to something that is not there has to be bad for us.

My children love games that involve chasing and being chased. My son's crew of eight-year-olds has developed a game of tag in which each person tagged becomes a zombie empowered to tag. This goes on until there is only one person left. The last person standing becomes the first zombie of the next game. They cannot get enough of it. And they always designate a safe zone for any player to retreat to if things get too intense and they need a breather. Yoga provides adults who need a breather from their endless game of leapfrog with a safe zone; it's called reality. To access this zone, we just need to align our mind with the present, bringing our awareness into this body, this breath, this moment.

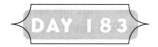

Genograms

I spent a year working at a substance-abuse unit in Cambridge, Massachu-setts. I was part of a team doctors, nurses, and counselors who had a week to ten days to provide a medically safe detox from whatever a patient was addicted to and to help them create a plan for their next steps on the road to recovery. As a counselor, one of my duties was to perform the intake interview once the patient was well enough to answer about an hour of questions. This interview was the first step in a comprehensive evaluation to help us understand how we could be of assistance. It was a responsibility that I took seriously. Professionals with twenty years of experience would be reading the results and forming their opinions in part based on what I had written. The first step in the interview process was to help the patient construct a genogram, specifying which individuals in her family tree had been addicts, which had been partnered with addicts, who had mental ill-ness, and any instances of trauma in the patient's life, from those inflicted by warfare to child abuse.

The effect this discussion had on both the person performing the inter-view and the patient was always transformational. Where there had been an isolated incident, a person needing medical help for an addiction, there was now the understanding of a larger pattern at work. I believe a genogram of any family's pattern of suffering due to contracted states—the addiction we all have to wanting this and not wanting that—would have the same effect. It would place our work on our mat and on our cushion into a larger, more informed context.

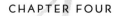

CHAPTER FOUR

173

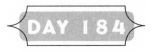

Scotch and Pall Malls

The symbols of my family's war with reality were Scotch and Pall Mall cigarettes. Whenever my mother's family got together, the adults would break out a deck of cards, Black Label beer, and Cutty Sark Scotch and chain-smoke filterless Pall Mall cigarettes all night. The kids would play unsupervised in another room as the voices around the card table slowly got louder and angrier.

The story that is written around this sort of scene is usually told along the lines of class, or ethnicity, or the family disease of addiction. I feel as though these perspectives catch the trees and miss the forest. Humanity is at war with reality. All of our other wars—the war on drugs, the war on poverty, the war on obesity, and the wars we have had with one another across the millennia—are just reflections of the war we are waging against having to live life on life's terms. Whether or not we think this sounds small and petty, or tragic and dreadful, it is the job that lies before us all. It is the calling that whispers to us in the midst of our contracted states to find peace, to bring peace, to make peace with this life we have been given.

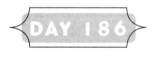

Making Peace

Because we are the ones who made war, only we can make peace. If we want to make progress, only we can take the first step. If we want amends to be made, we must be the ones to say we are sorry. If we want forgiveness, we must be the ones to forgive. If we want love, we must be the ones to say "I love you." If we want joy, we must be the ones who carry joy in our hearts. If we believe in yoga, we must be the ones who teach it through the way we live.

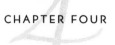

Nonreaction

The practice of *abhyasa* is transformative. In my own experience it has meant that I am now awake and paying attention. When I show up, you get my full attention. With *abhyasa* not only are we bringing all of our faculties to bear on the challenges and opportunities that fill our days, we are creating a momentum that eventually becomes a habit. The brain adapts to the priority of present-moment awareness. Over the years we begin to enjoy the benefits of a concentrated mind, the well-being it brings, and the excellence it facilitates. I am now able to move through my days without giving the power of my attention away to distractions, and as this ability has

CHAPTER FOUR

deepened, the amount of attention that I can pour into what matters has grown with it.

The practice of *vairagya*, or "renunciation," brings this process into the heart. The pull of the contracted states comes from our hearts' connection to them—we wish this person had loved us; we wish that person hadn't died; we wish we had done a better job—and each time we contract in this fashion we create a self who is not the self. We create a self who is just the daughter who could have been better. We create a self who is just the student who could have tried harder. *Abhyasa* lets us be right there as this is happening, *vairagya* teaches us to be with our experience without needing to coerce or abandon it. This readiness to be with our experience unconditionally allows us to learn about ourselves, one another, and how we can make better choices.

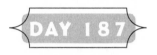

We See Things as We Are

From the contracted state of envy we see a world that justifies our envy. From the contracted state of anger we see a world that justifies our anger. From the contracted state of desire we see a world that justifies our desire. The contracted states are like colored lenses, changing the way we view the world. *Abhyasa* brings us into intimacy with our own felt experience and helps us to understand that making sound choices is very difficult when our options are viewed through the lens of a contracted state. Viewed through the lenses of victimhood and grievance, forgiveness feels like someone's idea of a sick joke. Viewed through the lens of shame, we are

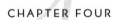

not worthy of another try at sobriety, so why not have a drink? We simply cannot let go, we cannot abide, and we will certainly never forgive. Being right there as we write these false narratives allows us to see how we create our own suffering.

We need a way to examine how we are seeing. We need enough space from our own thoughts to be able to see them more clearly. In ordinary consciousness we are like someone on the slopes of a mountain trying to determine its height and shape. The eyes that cannot take in the mountain at its base can understand that same mountain if they are brought to ten thousand feet. The practice of *vairagya* allows this perspective by teaching us to reflect on the mind rather than reacting to it.

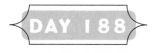

Not Reacting to Reacting

When people hear that "*vairagya*" means "nonreaction" they often assume that yoga practiced correctly therefore means an end to reacting. Maybe it does. That has not been my experience. *Vairagya* is the ability to allow our bodily sensations, thoughts, and feelings to arise and pass without getting caught up in them, without making a self out of them. *Abhyasa* has gotten us right there; *vairagya* gives us the ability to be the sky that holds the weather without being defined by that weather.

Getting started is the hard part. The months on our cushion come and go and there we are, right there, watching ourselves in one reaction after another, a human pinball machine lighting up and making weird noises at the slightest provocation. We develop two new contracted states. One is trying not to react to internal and external stimuli in meditation, the other is being upset with ourselves for having reacted to internal and external stimuli in meditation. Eventually, we realize that not reacting to the fact that we are reacting might be a great place to start.

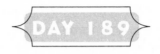

Changing Gears

For me, one of the most difficult contracted states is feeling like I am not enough. The premise of this state is that I am using yoga to be someone else because I am wrong the way I am—too much this and too little that—and that if I can just get this yoga thing right I will be a better person, a better husband, a better father. This state suggests that the person I need to be is not here yet. The wanting/striving I experience in this state makes any sort of intimacy with the present moment all but impossible. Once I understood the practice of *vairagya* and began to practice not reacting to my reactions, I began to take life a lot less personally. In particular, I started to take being me less personally. As I did so, the contracted state of feeling like I am not enough began to seem less and less relevant.

I began to practice being the sky that holds the weather. If the weather of anger is present, I am learning to hold anger with wisdom and compassion. If the weather of desire is present, I am learning to hold desire with wisdom and compassion. We are like a sky holding weather, not a sky fixing the fact of weather. The person I need to be is here, now, like a gear that I can shift into. I just need a little time and a little space to find that gear. The practice of *vairagya* creates the time and space to do so.

‹ DAY 190 ›

The Stone Wheel

Just as *abhyasa* turns the stone wheel of concentration until it is spinning with a self-sustaining momentum, *vairagya* turns the stone wheel of equanimity. As the wheel starts to turn, we begin to have moments when it is okay to have a feeling without reacting to it. We start to see that a feeling is a feeling, that sitting with this feeling is pretty much the same as sitting with that feeling. Our practice of nonreaction slowly expands to encompass a larger and larger range of feelings. We can sit with and acknowledge what it is to be with someone we love and just let that be so. We can sit with and acknowledge how much we miss someone and just let that be so. We begin to experiment with the feelings we have been afraid of, that have been disowned, that have become our shadow. We can sit with our deepest fears and grief and just let that be so. As this begins to happen we find that we can live without fear. Whatever arises in our internal and external world we can now meet with a calm faith—not certainty, just faith. We are arriving at the sort of equanimity that makes calm abiding, clear seeing, and right action possible.

CHAPTER FOUR

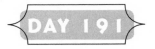

Impermanence

When a biological organism perceives something in its internal or external environment, it reacts. Those slow to react get eaten or starve. We carry this truth in every cell in our body. An aspect of that equation is that there is no time, no past, no future, only now. A shadow crosses the sun and the squirrels run for cover. A twig snaps and the deer stop and listen. No past, no future, only now. In meditation we watch this same pattern play out: the stimulus arises and the urge to react arises with it—the itch, the thought, the ache between the shoulders. If we sit with this play of sensations without reacting, something happens that offers us a genuine insight: the stimulus, the itch, the thought, the ache, arises, stays for a while, then passes. Things come and go. Good things, bad things, in-between things. They all come and go. Part of the space that we create through meditation in order to find an appropriate response is the knowledge that things change on their own and that it is okay to do nothing. The practice of *vairagya* brings us into the direct felt experience of impermanence and the infinity of choices that come with it.

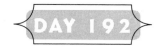

Sound

The discovery of impermanence, and our ability to bear witness to it as opposed to react to it, was a big deal for me. I had somehow made it to my late thirties without knowing that whatever I was feeling, seeing, having, not having, afraid of, or hoping for was about to change. This was huge, because it meant that I had permission to be still and to let things play out. I did not have to jump into every situation, every conversation, every opportunity. I was allowed to act wisely rather than impulsively.

It began as I listened to the sound of a bell fade into silence, watching form vanish. I was enthralled. I found a good blanket and an accommodating bench and sat in the cold listening to cars pass by on the country road in front of the retreat center where I was studying. The sound of a car would start out very faint; it would build, peak, fade, then vanish, the silence afterward holding the sounds of the forest, the creaking of the trees, the slight breeze. On the breeze drifted early spring, the smell of snow, earth, and leaves. The space between each passing car was a silent eternity of being, a perfect place to remember and to begin again.

CHAPTER FOUR

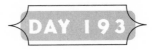

Remembering

Lost in a loop of action and reaction, we enter the realm of self-justification. Our actions make sense to us even if they don't make sense. To stay lost requires momentum, however. *Vairagya* arrests that momentum. We learn to pause and to enjoy the ability to pause. We learn to feel into the moment and to enjoy feeling into the moment. Sitting with something, being with something, starts to feel constructive. Music is the space between the notes—and we are learning to live in that space, to love its twilight rhythms, its whispers, and its truths. To find ourselves there is like coming home; to find ourselves there is to remember.

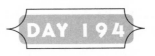

Pleasant and Unpleasant

My teachers begin with meditation on the body and the breath, then begin to include thoughts and feelings. The body and the breath are fairly soothing objects of meditation. Thoughts and feelings, not so much. The initial step toward addressing our thoughts and feelings is just to notice if they are pleasant, unpleasant, or neutral. I find that this is sustainable for about ten minutes; then I get bored and begin to suffer. I contract around toughing it out and that lasts for a couple of minutes. Returning to the body and the breath, things get pretty quiet again for a while. After a time I am ready to recommit to noticing whether my thoughts and feelings are pleasant, unpleasant, or neutral, but I keep the body and the breath in the background this time, noticing my thoughts and feelings but never losing touch with the rise and fall of my breathing, never losing touch with the way my body is a calm vibrant space. Without the full charge of my attention, thoughts and feelings flit about, then disappear. More and more of them are neutral; more and more often they aren't there at all. The bell rings and it is time to start walking meditation. As I get up I try staying in my body and my breath as I move toward the door.

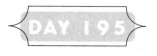

Continuity

For a while my teachers' encouragement that I bring continuity into my practice fell on deaf ears. I did not really know what they were talking about and it did not sound all that helpful, whatever it was. After a couple of years, however, I figured out what they were saying and within another couple of years began to try to follow their advice. The idea is that you work the technique you are being taught through the various moments of your day on retreat and once you get home. If you are learning to notice wanting and not wanting, you are noticing them while sitting, while walking, while eating, and while performing your chore. Sitting and waiting for the evening talk, you are noticing wanting and not wanting; standing in line for tea, you are noticing wanting and not wanting; and as you fall asleep, you are noticing wanting and not wanting. Once you get home, you are notic-

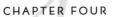

ing wanting and not wanting. You are practicing as if you believe it matters how wanting and not wanting show up in your life and as if you believe you can change your relationship to these primal habits of the mind.

I practice this way now and it feels like no big deal. It feels like what I came for. I wanted to learn this when I first started coming on retreats, but I did not know how. I did not know how to be responsible for my own learning. I thought just showing up would do the trick. Life respects us more than that. If we are going to learn the hardest thing there is to learn, it's not going to be by mistake. It's going to be a choice that we make and keep on making; it's going to be a choice that we practice with continuity.

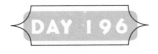

Sunday Morning in Manhattan

For a while I was teaching a yoga class in Manhattan at ten A.M. on Sunday mornings. The train ride in was a quiet affair, just the few unfortunates who had someplace to be on New York City's day of rest. After one of those rides I made my way across Union Square's temporarily abandoned park to the studio. I was about to cross Seventeenth Street when I heard an odd chirping sound. I looked to my right and saw that it came from an SUV moving so fast that it was rocking from side to side. The chirping sound was the squeal of its tires as they took the full weight of the vehicle, the other two tires catching air. As the SUV hurtled toward me, I noticed a police car in hot pursuit. The police had been so surprised to find themselves in a car chase on Sunday morning that their sirens weren't on, and with the exception of the chirping tires, the whole situation was unfolding in an odd, and potentially lethal, silence. They passed me as I stood in shock, then banked an extremely swift U-turn, hopping the curb, and charged back directly toward me. I ran like all the extras you have ever seen in any car chase in any movie. My arms were raised and I was screaming inarticulately. As I made my panicked way across Seventeenth Street, my meditation teachers would have been proud, because all I could think of was how sorry I was for the young people in the SUV that their lives had come to this. If I had died in that moment my last thought would have been the hope that they were going to be able to experience their eventual arrest as a turning point, that this chase would be the beginning of a better life for them. I had taken the practice of continuity off the cushion and into my heart.

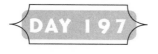

Steadiness

A year or two after I had integrated the concept of continuity into my practice I began to notice that my teachers on retreat kept using the term "steadiness," the ability to maintain your practice steadily, through highs and lows, choosing not to take the content of a given day personally. Not making a self out of rough going or smooth sailing, just applying the meditation technique of the day with continuity and steadiness.

Steadiness is an intention I set before I even show up on retreat, and one that I hold throughout. It is the intention to remember why I am there and who benefits from my practice, remember how fortunate I am to have the opportunity to practice, remember how countless individuals have gone their entire lives without one day of practice. Steadiness is holding those I practice with and for in my heart as I move from sitting to walking, walking to sitting. Steadiness is belief in the practice and belief in myself, and letting go of the rest.

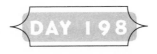

Being Steady

It has taken me decades of practice to unravel the fear I learned as a child from adults who reacted to each new occurrence in their lives as if it were the end of the world. As a parent it was one of the things I was extremely clear about not wanting to pass on to my children. The adults I grew up around had little or no faith in life. I wanted my children to learn to have faith in life from the way I met the normal ups, downs, and surprises it throws at all of us. I wanted to teach faith and self-confidence not with words but through living. I wanted to teach my children to be steady.

Teaching steadiness means being steady. But being steady happens only when we choose it and practice it. Eleven years into the actual practice of parenting, my children have come to expect me to be calm and steady. My wife has come to expect me to be calm and steady. My students have come to expect me to be calm and steady, and they are learning to be calm and steady teachers from my example. As my children meet life's ups and downs they are demonstrating their own version of steadiness because they have never seen anything else. The steadiness I put out into the world comes back to me, and I am nourished and sustained by the steadiness of those around me. Being steady spreads.

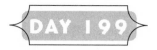

Continuity and Steadiness

Mindfulness begins with *abhyasa* and *vairagya* and progresses into a detailed study of what is true in every area of our lives. Whether we are studying the sensations of the body, the breath, or our thoughts and feelings, we are learning to be right there with an open heart and an open mind, seeking only to know what is true here and now. The techniques of mindfulness amount to an intention that we hold to steadily and apply with continuity. It is a grown-up practice that prepares us for a grown-up life. We find that if we can be right there for the breath, we can be right there for everything else. We find that if we can be the sky that holds the weather of our thoughts and feelings, we can be the sky that holds the people in our life as they experience their own thoughts and feelings. We find that if we can be steady in our practice, we can be steady in our life. We find that if we can practice principle with continuity in yoga, we can practice principle with continuity in life.

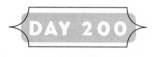

A Water Park

It happened at a water park in Pennsylvania. I was holding my newborn son, Dylan, and my wife, Mariam, was in a wading pool with our three-year-old daughter, Jasmine. They were holding hands and laughing. Mariam looked up at me and smiled; I smiled back. We had made it. We had become a family.

Mariam had been born ready to be part of a family; I had not. My wiring had not been developed or was just not there, but in either case I did not know how to share my life, my time, my heart. Growing up, I had needed to be iron to survive, but that was no longer true and I did not know how to be anything else. Mindfulness taught me to start by reflecting on being iron rather than living from it. This created enough space for my family to fit into my life, to form a wedge and open my heart. On tiny copies of my feet, my children ran up the iron steps to my heart.

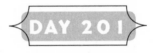

What Holds the Sky?

Any time spent with our own felt experience reveals a wounded heart, a heart with issues that do not feel as if they can ever be resolved, losses, grievances, wounds, and regrets that feel like more than we can hold. The practice of opening the mind reveals the need to reopen our hearts. Just as there is a practice to return the mind to its original nature and purpose, so too is there a practice of the heart that returns it to its true nature and purpose. Free the mind and it becomes the sky that can hold the weather of our lives, but what holds the sky? A heart that is free.

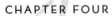

THREE WAYS TO ESTABLISH MINDFULNESS

1) Stop and move from thinking to feeling for a few breaths throughout the day. Keep coming back to your body and your breath until it becomes part of how you enjoy life. Then do what you enjoy.

2) Work up to practicing mindfulness meditation for at least thirty minutes a day. The figure I shoot for is three to six hours of meditation a week, and thirty minutes each day gets you there. It takes a lot of effort to get that stone wheel moving, but you will find that it is a lot easier to keep that wheel spinning than to get it started.

3) Spend time each year in the company of mindfulness teachers supported by a mindfulness community.

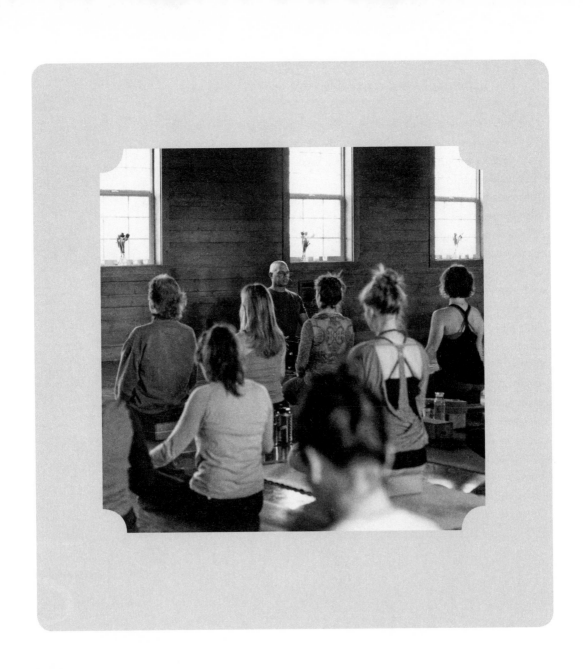

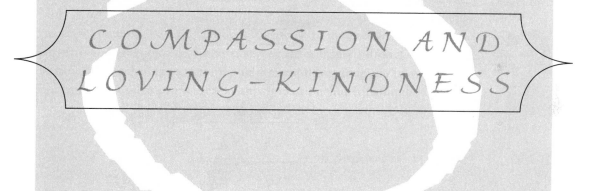

CHAPTER FIVE

COMPASSION AND
LOVING-KINDNESS

Section 1.33 of the Yoga Sutras outlines the *brahmaviharas*, the four divine states, pioneered by the Buddha as necessary counterparts to the practice of mindfulness. They are the four virtues we practice to develop our hearts so that they can hold the world that is revealed by mindfulness with kindness, compassion, joy, and equanimity. They allow us to cultivate a steady mind and a steady heart, a spacious mind and a spacious heart, a mind that understands and a heart that knows, a mind that lets go and a heart that forgives.

The *brahmaviharas* are the practices of loving-kindness, compassion, joy, and equanimity. The next two chapters will be dedicated to these practices and to exploring how they work as a practical system for living and loving well, building effortlessly on the work we have already done with the *yamas*, *niyamas*, and mindfulness.

My teachers have taught me the practices of the *brahmaviharas* as loving-kindness, compassion, joy, and equanimity, in that order, but I will be tweaking the sequence of the essays to reflect my own process. I had to arrive at compassion before loving-kindness was something I could practice without falling into the contracted state of codependency. I needed to practice equanimity before I could move into the true abundance that is the practice of joy, and it is with joy that I share these practices with you. Together we will remember that each of us has a heart so spacious that it can hold the world just as we find it. Together we will remember that each of us has a heart so full that it can pour love into everything we do and everyone we meet without ever becoming empty.

Compassion

A few years ago I went on a ten-day meditation retreat in California's Yucca Valley. It was very well attended, and each morning I sat at the back of a large room full of people as they enjoyed a brief opportunity to ask questions at what was otherwise a silent gathering. Early on I recognized a pattern: every day when it was time for questions someone would raise her hand and say she was having trouble with judgment of herself and judgment of others. Because I was having a lot of trouble with everything, it took me a while to see how much pain there was in the room due to the mental phenomenon people were calling judgment, but eventually it sunk in. When people start watching the mind, they start seeing how much suffering our mental habit of judging ourselves and others is causing.

The leaders of the retreat seemed to think so as well, so on the fourth afternoon they dedicated a practice session to forgiving ourselves for being imperfect, for making mistakes, and for having to learn about life by living it. This was a flexion point in my understanding of the aim of spiritual practice. For much of the previous two decades I had thought I was healing from the results of my toxic relationship with myself, but it had not occurred to me to actually address the relationship itself. Me, and my story, were just a fact of life—like gravity—and spiritual practice was about making the best of it.

That afternoon on retreat I came to understand that the judgment we inflict upon the world is a reflection of the judgment we inflict upon ourselves, and that if we want relief from constantly judging the world around us we must learn to stop judging ourselves. The practice of forgiveness has taught me that there is a difference between a person and a behavior. A behavior can be unforgivable, but the troubled, pained, confused individual who acts out the behavior is not.

My teachers did not try to teach me to forgive others. They taught me to see that it made sense to forgive myself and to let go of the past. I now see forgiveness as a primary life skill. Adults need the skill of forgiveness if we are to have sustainable relationships and communities. And self-forgiveness is only the beginning. Once we learn to forgive ourselves for being human we are able to accept the humanity of others. We will be less and less troubled by the inability of human beings to avoid mistakes and their penchant for acting imperfectly. We will be able to hold space for others as they go through the sacred learning process of a human lifetime. We will desire the calm abiding energy of compassion and see how offering it to others is a way of honoring ourselves.

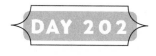

Mary Ann

Just as I was turning fifty, my birth mother, Mary Ann, contacted me for the first time in many years. I had been in touch with her sixteen years before, and we had met but had fallen out of contact. She wrote that she had waited for as long as she could for me to reach out to her, but could wait no longer and felt compelled to reach out herself. It was inconvenient. I had a lot going on, and returning to an ancient pain was not high on my to-do list. It got worse: I demanded an explanation for why she had abandoned me, and I got one. The white mother of a brown child, she told me how her family and her church had abandoned her. I had languished for two years in an orphanage in my hometown while my grandparents refused to visit. As far as I know, they never met their own grandchild because he was brown. The Catholic orphanage's policy was not to place brown children in families, so at twenty my mom was on her own in her attempts to get me placed in a loving home.

My back went out and I could not surf or practice asana. Things were bad. Then my training kicked in. I knew my ethical commitments dictated a loving response no matter what. I knew to align behind that response and to be content to do so. I had strong reserves of momentum carrying me forward toward that response from years of practice. I had the capacity to reflect on feeling like a victim rather than live from it, which gave me the inner space to attempt compassion. The practice of compassion has taught me to put myself in another person's shoes. Mary Ann's family had abandoned her. My adopted family had never abandoned me. Mary Ann's church had abandoned her. My spiritual communities had been, and were being, impeccable supports in my life. I thought about my children, who have had a wonderful experience of extended family, and of how I was sure that they would embrace my birth mom. I thought about how Mary Ann needed to know that things had worked out for me. Her church might have abandoned her, but God had not abandoned us. I invited her for a visit and she said yes.

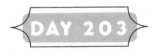

Forgiveness Is Practical

Early on in the practice of mindfulness we discover deep-seated conflicts with what has been going on. We don't like what he did, we really don't like what she did, we don't like the way that went down, we can't understand why those people are the way they are, we don't even like how we are handling our meditation practice. All in all, things could be going better, and while we hope that someday in the future we will be less judgmental about the way things are, we are also aware of our track record. When we hear

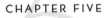

about forgiveness we get glimpses of an entirely different way of relating to the most challenging emotional situations in our lives, but when we try it for ourselves we usually run up against the fact that what someone did, or what we did, was just plain wrong. Forgiveness does not seem practical in this instance. Mindfulness reveals the unhappiness and turmoil that our inability to forgive causes us. We come to see that although it sometimes appears impossible, forgiveness would be a practical solution to some of the greatest suffering in our lives. We realize that resentments are a form of bondage and that forgiveness can offer freedom. We begin to soften and become ready to try.

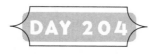

Meeting Pain with Compassion

For a long time, my teachers suggested that I meet pain with compassion. This sounded pious and unrealistic to me, but eventually I came to understand that they were not talking about walking the streets to find people to help but about dealing with my own pain. Mindfulness reveals a tremendous amount of human suffering, in both our own lives and in the lives of those around us. My teachers were showing me that the first step toward addressing suffering is to develop the habit of compassion, and that I should begin by facing the pain that was closest at hand—my own. I had learned to be right there as I began an in-breath, had a thought, or experienced a feeling. Meeting what happened next with compassion felt like a powerful way to turn yoga into action.

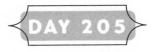

Acknowledge, Accept, Understand

I was taught three steps to meeting pain with compassion. First, we must become willing to acknowledge that suffering is present. Second, we must remove our resistance to it, by progressing to an attitude of acceptance. The final step is one of investigation, with the intention to learn and to understand. It might seem simple enough, but it is usually the last thing we want to do when we are suffering. So instead we begin with something small, something simple. We sit and try to be right there with each breath, and when the mind wanders we meet our wandering mind with compassion. Once the moment has passed we return to being right there at the beginning of the in-breath.

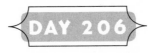

Returning to the Anchor

My teachers taught me to train my mind by bringing it to what they call an "anchor." The anchor is where you aim your attention. It can be the beginning of the in-breath or the sound of birds in a tree nearby. It can be the felt experience of awareness itself, but it is specific and does not change during the course of a period of meditation. As you can imagine, focusing your attention on something specific and trying not to let it waver is a vexingly difficult task. Every couple of breaths your mind drifts, usually to something you have thought about over and over again and are sick and tired of. Not only have you failed at staying right there, you are boring yourself to death with your repetitive petty grievances, fears, and desires. Suffering is in the house.

When learning to concentrate, this moment of drifting is met with a simple and effective statement: "Not now." Then you return to your anchor, refining your ability to align and repeatedly realign with the present moment in the form of the anchor. In the practice of mindfulness a new opportunity presents itself. Once you have recognized that you are no longer at your anchor you can meet your wandering mind with compassion, acknowledging and accepting that it has wandered, before returning to your anchor. Finding the ability to acknowledge and accept the reality of the moment you are in before returning to your anchor. Learning that ability with the body, the breath, the mind, and the heart.

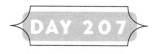

Acknowledging That Suffering Is Present

Denying that suffering is present has a couple of practical purposes. If we do not acknowledge it, we do not have to feel it. If we do not acknowledge it, we do not need to do anything about it. At least, that is, until the consequences of denial start to outweigh the benefits. We cannot choose when that moment is for another person, but asana, *pranayama*, and meditation can help us choose for ourselves. Being around people who are choosing the truth helps too.

One of the challenges we face as we learn the practice of compassion is that we tend to both underestimate and overestimate its importance. We think it is really not that big a deal and want to skip it to get to the bigger issues, and we also think that it will open the floodgates to a grief, an anger, a weakness, an attraction, a something that is too great to bear. The truth lies somewhere in between. The simple acknowledgment of suffering shifts the energy of a situation, changing the way we perceive it as well as the paths that lead from it. The Buddha said that once we know something to be true we must live up to it. There is power in knowing something to be true, and we choose that power for ourselves when we acknowledge that suffering is present.

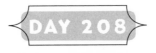

Wanting Things to Be Okay

One of the reasons I resist acknowledging suffering in my life is that I just want things to be okay. I know that love is possible. I know that skillful living is possible. And I know the harmony and joy that come when those two possibilities are brought together. It all seems so simple: let's just do that, have that, be that, and not worry about anything else. And life shrugs.

My wanting everything to be okay amounts to a contracted state in which only certain parts of life are welcomed and others are met with aversion. As I acknowledge this habit of mine to have preferences, to become attached to them, and to act foolishly when I am influenced by them, my heart softens toward the many people in my life I have judged for being like me. As my heart softens around my own and other people's behavior, everything starts to feel workable—everything starts to feel okay.

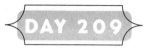

Aversion

Before I can do anything about the suffering in my life I have to acknowledge it as it is without judgment or wishing things were other than they are. The practice of meeting pain with compassion begins with learning to acknowledge that this is where we are now, thinking, "This is what jealousy is like," or "This is what doubt is like." In the space provided by mindfulness we learn to acknowledge the habits of our mind without making a self out of them. I am not an angry person; I am simply having the experience of anger like everyone else who has ever lived. And we can learn about ourselves and everyone else if we stay just a little longer right there with what it is to contract around a fear or a desire.

To understand the power of this we must consider the problem of meeting pain with aversion. This reaction to pain is so ingrained that we do not know that it is a habit of the mind that can be changed. It feels entirely normal to meet the unpleasant with aversion. And it is, but so are the protracted bouts of mind-made suffering that come when we resist life as opposed to working with it. When we meet life with aversion we keep it at arm's length, holding at bay all that a situation could teach us. We become like someone on a plane stuck on the runway, cramped and uncomfortable without any of the benefits. Then we remember our training and soften around the felt experience of aversion. Taking a breath, we say, "Oh, this is what aversion is like."

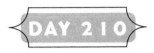

Receiving the Truth

We cannot give to someone who is unwilling to receive. Neither can life. To acknowledge the truth is to receive what life has to offer and to be willing to start there. This is a way of living that can bring peace into all of our relationships, be they with food, money, health, sex, intoxicants, other people, power, art, or our careers. Our relationship to an entire range of mental and emotional states, and to ourselves, can proceed within an atmosphere of gracious acknowledgment that what is being given is all that needs to be given to achieve the highest good for all. It begins by being right there with our breath and, when our mind wanders, meeting our wandering mind with compassion.

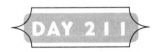

An Embodied Practice of Compassion

Yoga is an embodied practice. In mindfulness we learn to feel into what is true and to live from that truth. The heart virtues are felt into as well. To acknowledge a truth we have held at arm's length is an action that includes our mental, emotional, and physical bodies. To acknowledge something is to allow it into our consciousness, into our heart. This is above all else a felt experience, and yoga teaches us to be right there for it.

Acknowledging the presence of suffering is the first step. It brings our suffering into the open space of our awareness, where we can begin to see and feel into it. One of the first things we perceive about suffering is that we do not like it and that we want it to go away. The energy of not wanting our suffering is a well-practiced contracted state that perpetuates the original suffering while adding an additional layer of its own—one of judgment and craving. To take the charge out of this predicament, we need to learn to meet our suffering with acceptance. To meet the contracted state of not wanting with the relaxed body, deep slow breath, spacious mind, and open heart that are available to us when we move into acceptance.

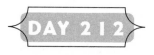

DAY 212

An Obstructed View

When I talk about meeting pain with compassion in a workshop setting I hold up my hand like a police officer gesturing for oncoming traffic to stop. I say that this is how we usually respond to pain. We say, "No," we say, "Stop." I point out that when my hand is in front of my face I cannot see what is in front of me. All I can see is the back of my hand. All I can see is my resistance. I then shift my hand so that it is palm up. I say this is acceptance. It is not resignation; it is accepting something so that we can see what it's all about. I show how I can now see my palm and the space around my palm. Where there was an obstructed view there is now clear open space.

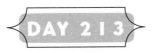

Judgment

The premise of meeting pain with compassion is that we have already tried meeting it with judgment. We have judged a situation to be unacceptable and this judgment is making things worse. Where we had a situation on our hands, we now have a situation *and* the suffering our judgment of the situation is causing. It's become a bit of a mess. Are we angry because of the situation or are we angry because of our judgment about the people in the situation? Are we afraid of the situation or are we afraid of our projections about what would happen if we failed? We reflexively judge the present based on a set of beliefs in a life moving so fast we often don't have a chance to reflect on how those beliefs worked out for us last time. Instead, habits of mind that are outdated or just unworthy of us get rolled out in situation after situation, and the suffering they cause obscures their role in the confusion they are sowing.

Time spent right there with the body and the breath settles us down and gets us used to being settled. The disruption our reflexive judgments are causing us starts to become noticeable. Connected to our bodies and our hearts, we are starting to feel the harm our habitual judgments create for ourselves and others. Our focus shifts from what we are doing to how we are being, and we begin to seek a mental settling to match the physical and emotional settling we are learning on our mat and our cushion. We are beginning to wonder, "Why all the fuss?" Maybe if we could just accept that she is like she is, that I am like I am, that the traffic is like it is, maybe if we could accept this, whatever "this" is, things wouldn't be so hard. Maybe peace is something we can choose after yoga the way we have learned to choose it in yoga.

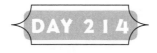

Reversing the Flow

Eckhart Tolle speaks eloquently about the suffering we create for ourselves by saying no to this moment. The moment is an expression of all that is, and our rejection isn't going to change anything except our experience of it. Despite its futility, and the pain it causes, our war with reality is all we have known. It is a pain we have practiced. Meeting that pain with compassion turns a problem into an opportunity. In meditation, the mind wanders from its anchor every couple of breaths, providing us with numerous opportunities to acknowledge, accept, and eventually learn from things not going our way. In everyday life, we contract around our rejection of what is with almost as much regularity as the mind wanders in meditation. Meeting our no with compassion reverses the flow of energy in a moment. Where we had been working against life, we can begin to work with it.

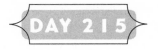
Acceptance

I lost my sister Wendy before I had a yoga practice. She died in the winter, and the following spring, as I was celebrating my first year of sobriety, I began driving to Wellesley College to run around a pond that lives there. I'd go there alone and walk from the parking lot to the water's edge. The run is a little more than two miles around on a dirt path surrounded by trees and never more than a few feet from the water. I'd run around the pond for an hour or so, finding a rhythm, then letting go into it. I liked the way the dust of the path rose up to cover my running shoes and my ankles. I liked the way the rhythm of the run and the rhythm of my breathing merged. I liked the way I became the forest and the pond, running and crying for someone who died from a broken heart. I liked the way the pond and the forest helped me to feel what I was feeling.

When I was done I would walk to the car and back to a life I did not agree with. I did not agree with finding my sister dead from an overdose at thirty-one. I did not agree with the way her lips and fingernails were blue or the way it felt worse than death to have the enormity of what I was experiencing be so undeniable, so immutable. I did not agree to my powerlessness or to the fact that I was having this experience alone, knowing I would always bear it alone because my sister was dead. I did not agree with my life the way anyone who is in grief does not agree with her life. And as I approached my car I could feel myself recommitting to life anyway. I could feel the way my heart was turning toward the future I was living into with the courage of acceptance.

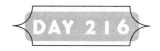

Future Suffering

Acceptance is a redirection of the energy of a situation. Doors that were closed open, understandings arrive unbidden, relationships heal and end. There is a watershed quality to this moment, a sense that things have changed in ways that will be revealed only in the fullness of time. Acceptance is a slight shift in the way we are sitting, a slowing and deepening of the breath, an inclination of the mind from what we are against to what we are for. It is both the grand gesture and the softening of the face as we move from thinking to feeling.

I love the ability of asana, *pranayama*, and meditation to teach us the subtle side of acceptance: the refinement of how we are aiming our attention, the awakening and softening that follows awareness. This aspect of our practice allows us to notice the acorn of resistance before it becomes an oak tree, the inner realignment replacing the grand gesture. Future suffering avoided with a deepening of the breath and a decision to wait and see.

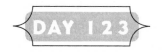

To Acknowledge and to Accept

My children came into the world with the understanding that nature is delightful and worthy of our undivided attention, every animal an adventure, every detail worth committing to memory. Countless conversations began with "Did you know that . . . ?" Some of my favorites were about animals doing extraordinary things. The orangutan who bribed a neighboring ape with treats to gain access to the wire he needed to pick his lock and escape his cage at night. Or the aquarium octopus that went on nightly raids of other tanks without anyone's realizing.

In each case, the people caring for these animals had no idea what could possibly be happening. Nothing in their experience prepared them for the truth. For them to arrive at an accurate understanding of their situation it was necessary for them to first acknowledge that something outside of what they considered possible was happening. It was only once they acknowledged and accepted what they did not know that they became available to the truth.

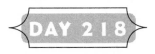

Getting off a Boat

As the practice of concentration—aligning and realigning to the present moment—progresses to mindfulness, we are taught various techniques that help us to begin investigating the habits of our mind. One such technique is bringing our attention to the breath or the body as an anchor, and when it moves away treating this moving away as if your mind had gotten on a boat and drifted off. Once you realize that you have left the anchor you are working with and are on a boat, the technique is to name the boat (for example: "desire" or "aversion"), then return to the anchor. Within a day or so most students using this technique have a sense of which boats their minds prefer, what patterns there are, and where their minds habitually go.

The moment of recognition that we are on a boat is actually a priceless opportunity for both insight and developing compassion as a reflex. The understanding that our mind is floating away on pretty much the same boats all of the time, day after day, can be a little deflating, but it also gives us a sense of where the focus of our practice should be, of what areas of our lives are out of balance or unresolved. We react to discovering that we are on a boat the way we habitually react when things aren't going our way. Meeting that moment with compassion lays the groundwork for bringing compassion into some of the most difficult areas of our lives. Learning to acknowledge that we are on a boat and to accept it before naming the boat. Pausing, not rushing, as we acknowledge, then soften to accept what is before we get off the boat.

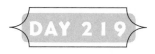

Mirroring

When I was working with adolescents, my help was not always well received. There were times of sublime connection and mutual growth, and then there were times when I was being yelled at as if asking someone not to eat in the living room were a crime against humanity. The children I cared for attacked with such vehemence that an untrained adult would be left speechless. After a while I discovered a way to respond to this kind of attack that maintained my authority and my intention to teach, yet managed to uplift. I would simply explain to the child that she was being rude, as if she were unaware of her behavior. It was comical and effective. A seventeen-year-old would swear at me at the top of her lungs, and I would take a breath and then calmly say, "Sarah, you are being rude. Let's try that again," as if being rude had not been her intention. No matter how mad the child was, it got through to her. She knew I was going to stick to my guns, that I would stay professional and stay connected to her no matter what she said. It left her with no reason to continue treating me rudely. She might continue for a while to save face, but the moment had passed.

This is the transformative power of meeting pain with compassion, the practice of acknowledging the difficult, the unpleasant, the scary, and the tedious and greeting it with acceptance. The situation remains, life is still life, but it has become workable.

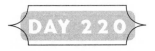

DAY 220

Galileo

I use the story of Galileo's life to teach the practice of mindfulness and compassion. I begin by saying that his first great contribution to human understanding was to say, "I don't know." Rather than trusting the accepted wisdom of his day, he admitted that he did not understand how the planets moved and spent a protracted period of time ardently watching the arising and passing of the stars, which led to a far more accurate sense of the solar system and Earth's place in it.

I make the case that the yoga student is a modern Galileo. Acknowledging and accepting what we do not know, we watch the arising and passing of internal and external stimuli to gain a more accurate sense of the world we live in and our place in it. Galileo's story demonstrates the flow from practice to understanding. Mindfulness brings us to the point of acknowledging and accepting what is true here, now. Acknowledging and accepting what is true opens up an opportunity for learning and eventually understanding. The name for this sort of understanding in Sanskrit is "*prajna*," or "wisdom"—a wisdom that has developed momentum.

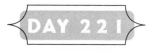

Prajna

Yoga sets off a chain reaction of awareness and understanding in our lives. First, our bodies start to feel better. We have more energy; our perspective becomes more positive, more hopeful. We begin to unravel cause and effect. We find that on days when we meditate or pray things go more smoothly. We make a decision at work that reflects something we learned on our yoga mat, and it yields positive results.

Initially, we experience these insights separately, but over time we begin to see that they are part of a larger process of awakening that is happening in our lives because of yoga. The books we read, the people we meet, the doors that open, the doors that close all start to feel like aspects of a process whose aim is our growth. Like a person climbing a mountain, each step on the path allows us to see and to understand a little more. *Prajna* is the understanding that wisdom is a process.

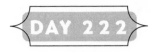

Being Curious

To acknowledge and accept the moment connects us to it. We are right there with all five senses awake to what is, and it is often enough just to rest in our felt experience of being here. Much of life appears to exist simply to be appreciated. My dog, Chelsea, is like that: her purpose is the experience of being Chelsea and eating pizza crust. Mindfulness is concerned with suffering and the end of suffering, something that much of life is empty of. Then we contract around a situation and we are back to work acknowledging and accepting that we are in a contraction. Once this has happened there is a precious moment when appreciation can become curiosity. What just happened? Why contract around wanting this or not wanting that? Why numb out and drift away now?

We think yoga will require us to gain special skills and powers. This is not the case. Yoga simply trains us to use the special skills and powers we already have. One of them is the wisdom we acquire once we have learned to be curious, like a child examining everything, or like an adult who studies the way she is choosing to see something, someone, or herself.

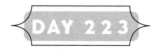

The Heart Softens

The first chapter of the Yoga Sutras lays out a foundation for spiritual practice. The practices we are taught to embrace consist of learning to see and learning to be. The mindfulness practices teach us how to see; the *brahmaviharas*—the practice of loving-kindness, compassion, joy, and equanimity—teach us how to be. These two practices form a perfect circle. As we learn to see we are moved to be, and as we find authentic being we are moved to see.

The link between seeing and being is the heart. True seeing touches the heart and authentic being expresses it. In a contraction, we see only that which confirms what we already believe. To acknowledge and to accept that we are in a state of contraction changes how we are standing in the world. The body begins to soften and the heart begins to open as we start to see and be. Becoming curious, we open our eyes a little more, take in a little more, understand a little more. Life as a problem slowly returns to just being life, and the heart softens a little more.

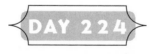

Forgiveness

Right there with our own felt experience we discover that we are living like we are characters in a movie, waiting for the big moment when suddenly our lives make sense. But the movie has lasted decades and the audience is becoming restless. Some of what we are waiting for does not exist. Some of what we are waiting for will never come. And some of what we are waiting for only we can give ourselves.

Acknowledging and accepting this state of affairs for what it is, we become curious. We were born to see and to understand, so we do. We see what cannot ever exist. We see what will never come. But most of all, we see what we must become willing to give to ourselves. Forgiveness.

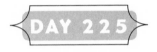

No Hatred

It is breathtaking to realize that human anger amounts to anger at ourselves that we project onto the world and onto one another. That how we treat Earth is a reflection of how we treat our bodies, that how we treat one another is a reflection of how we treat ourselves. Unable to manage the experience of the self we have created, permanently disturbed by what we have or have not done, we attack anything we see that reminds us of our own disowned shadow. Without this identification there would be no hatred.

Now imagine the possibility of resolving our relationship to ourselves, a process that ends not in perfection but in acknowledgment, acceptance, and understanding. Imagine if there were no one to hate.

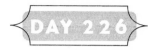

Self-forgiveness

I began the process of forgiving myself with no sense of the effect it would have on my life. I was five days into a very well-led and effective meditation retreat and I was in the zone. It was an afternoon sitting session and we were being taught to review our lives in ten-year increments. Decade by decade, we allowed an unresolved moment or unskillful behavior to come to us and then offered ourselves forgiveness for being imperfect, making mistakes, and having to learn about life through living it.

As I went through the decades of my life I was able to really feel back into who I was in that life moment. I could see and feel the level of confusion and pain that accompanied my unskillful behavior. I saw how ignorant I was of what I could only know by living longer, by being *me* longer. I saw how if I had known then what I know now I would have chosen differently. I saw how I had confused the person with the behavior. The person I met in these time-traveling meditations was always doing the best he could with the hand he thought he had been dealt, and that I could forgive.

CHAPTER FIVE

5

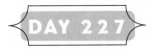

Letting Myself Off the Hook

The point of mindfulness is for us to be able to see what is true, and this certainly happened for me as I went back and looked at moments in my life when I had acted unskillfully. I had been holding myself accountable to an unfair set of criteria and had been planning to do so indefinitely. I had unresolved grievances with myself and they were going to stay that way. I should have known better, been better, been less, been more, been someone else somewhere else, and that was that. I should never have been me! The unfairness and absurdity of the way I was standing in judgment of myself landed. It was not credible and it was not in any way grounded in the truth of my actual experience of life.

In the calm, still environs of the meditation retreat I set my burden down. I let myself off the hook because it made sense to do so. It felt good, it felt mature, it felt like acknowledging, accepting, and understanding the life that had brought me here. In the days that followed on the retreat, we began the work of forgiving others and the same dynamic was revealed to be at play as I judged others. But it was different. Once I had let myself off the hook there was no charge around letting others off the hook. When we are on the hook we look and point and say, "Why isn't she on a hook? Look at her." When we are off the hook we don't really care about hooks, don't even believe in them, much less want to put someone else on one. When I let myself off the hook everyone else came off with me.

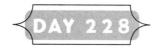

Making the Case

Part of the excellence of the instruction I received in how to forgive myself was that it used the mechanism that gets us stuck to get us unstuck. We make a case for not forgiving ourselves with a rudimentary sort of logic in which things are either right or wrong. "Lying is wrong, I lied, I should never have lied, therefore I am wrong." In the court of self-esteem there is no statute of limitations; once you are wrong you stay wrong.

The practice I was taught engages that part of our belief system directly. It asks:

YOGA: Do you have the right to be imperfect?

THE CRITIC: Well ... yes, of course you do.

YOGA: Do you have the right to make mistakes?

THE CRITIC: Well ... yes, everyone knows that.

YOGA: Do you have the right not to know things and to learn?

THE CRITIC: Yes, you do....

YOGA: If this is so, is it not wrong to judge yourself for these things?

THE CRITIC: ...Yes.

YOGA: Should you allow yourself to be imperfect, make mistakes, and learn?

THE CRITIC: Yes, I should. [*sigh*] But, yoga, what shall I do now?

YOGA: You must forgive yourself with at least as much regularity as you have been condemning yourself.

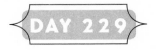

Being Imperfect

Eckhart Tolle teaches that once we lose touch with our true nature we create a mind-made self that lives with a perpetual sense of being partial and precarious. This partial and precarious self bears a strong resemblance to Einstein's mind-made prison, and I would add that shortly after we form it we become obsessed with perfection. We start to think that if we could only be perfect, this pervasive sense that we, and our surroundings, are not enough would go away. All I want is the perfect body, bank account, love, success, house, friends, children, health, car, garden, asana practice, and everything and anything else I have forgotten; is that so wrong? One of the flies in the champagne of life is that we keep being imperfect. It is really too much. I just cannot get over the way I keep messing up my perfect world.

A belief is a thought we keep thinking until it becomes a habit. It is quite an experience to feel what is on the other side of our unconscious assumption that we should be perfect. There is no need to try to imagine it or get it right; we just have to practice forgiving ourselves for being imperfect. Before long we will mean it.

CHAPTER FIVE

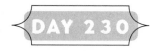

The Possibility of Beauty

Each of us has a knack for something. Men are supposed to be good at a lot of things I am horrible at. I don't really do cars, woodwork, painting, fixing, or handiness in general. I am not bad at putting together IKEA stuff, which makes me think I am not a total loss, but it was not until I hit my twenties that I discovered something I had a real knack for. I first noticed it patrolling at night in the mountain phase of ranger school. In circumstances that amounted to a very cold hell I started to notice how the mountain ranges were shaped and how the outline of those shapes could be picked out against the nighttime sky. The shape of each mountain was utterly unique, providing those who cared to look with landmarks as pronounced as street signs. I was never lost in the mountains because the shape of each mountain was something I could understand like a language. In the frozen hardship of ranger school I discovered that I had an eye for terrain.

Once I became aware of this skill, I realized that I had always had it. At an early age the camps and schools I attended were mini landscapes, the details of which had felt sweet and familiar to me. After ranger school I was stationed in Germany and spent the next three years roaming Europe using a topographical map. Before traveling anywhere I would spend days savoring the details of the landscape I was about to enter. Everywhere you go is beautiful if you have an eye for terrain. The beauty lies in the endless series of unique juxtapositions. This river runs close to town here, then gets narrow by this field. This high ground becomes steep, then levels off, creating a meadow from which you can see that valley below. The surface of the earth is an endless poem that unfolds as each imperfect shape connects perfectly to the next. To love the surface of the earth is to love the perfect imperfection of the world—and to know that imperfection is the possibility of beauty.

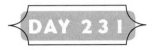

Standing Up Where We Have Fallen Down

Once you become aware of the world around you, you realize that everything in it is completely and equally unique. Everything that we will encounter in this lifetime has never been before and will never be again. You can see this in how every line runs its own course, whether it is the line that is the Alps or the line that is the edge of a leaf. The line that is our life is like this too. What makes our life unique is where we fall down and where we rise up again. That's what makes our line so special, because no one else can get up where we have fallen down. Only we can.

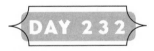

Forgiving Ourselves for Being Imperfect

Life seems to come at us all at once. We form a self, get a few priorities together, and come out swinging. Many of the critical details are missing and time is always short. In a best-case scenario we are a work in progress on a speeding train. In the worst case that train is headed nowhere fast. We are born into as many forms of suffering as there are stars in the sky and still we do the best we can with what we have. If the human experience could be summed up in one sentence, it would be "She dragged herself out of the hell she was born into to create a better life for her children." So, yeah, I think humans should forgive themselves for being imperfect. I think it's the least we can do. And it's also the best we can do.

In addition to forgiveness being the only sane response to the human condition, there is the truth of the ever-changing nature of reality to take into account. Nature does perfect as process, as change, as diversity, as a riot of color, as the predator and the prey. We do perfect as process as well, and the process is not over yet.

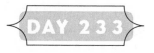

Making Mistakes

We live in a time when Western science is making significant contributions to our understanding of the practices of mindfulness and compassion. Researchers are telling us that to have an extra-ordinary response when something outside of the ordinary happens is a key part of how we grow, both individually and collectively. Our maps of reality are refined and rewritten when we reach their edges and bump up against the unexpected. This is our natural reaction to making a mistake. It is innately human, and adding suffering to the process misses the point.

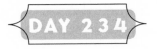

The Charge

Our reaction to making a mistake is in part a result of the way the brain is designed. It wants to learn more, and if something unexpected happens, this indicates that there is more to know about reality. Children love surprises and learning new things about their world, but adults have to work at it. As adults we burden ourselves with the expectation that we should not make mistakes. There is a special sort of anger that I reserve for those times when I mess up. I have a moment of speechless rage and instead of learning I get lost in aversion. This is not skillful. While my brain is trying to focus on what *is happening* my mind is focusing on what *should not have happened*. This makes things confusing and I usually make another mistake as a result.

The practice of meeting pain with compassion has given me a skillful way to navigate a difficult situation. At times of great possibility and learning I am often in a place of extreme contraction. Learning to acknowledge and accept what is happening as a matter of course, as a practiced way of being, allows me to move through reaction and into learning.

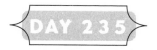

Forgiving Ourselves for Being Learners in This Lifetime

Forgiving myself for being imperfect and making mistakes was cathartic. Forgiving myself for being a learner in this lifetime took some processing. At first, I couldn't figure out what my teachers were getting at. There is a special form of mortification that happens when we start learning something new. We do the math and realize how many mistakes we would not have made if we knew "this" ten years ago. One of my regrets about getting sober at twenty-six is that I went through college in an alcoholic bottom. In my late twenties I knew a number of young people who got sober in their teens and were sober throughout their college years. Their complaints about not fitting in at the frat parties fell on deaf ears as I imagined all the pain I would have skipped and all the connection and meaning I would have experienced instead. Eventually I learned to appreciate the power of that pain and how it taught me to appreciate sobriety when it did come. Eventually I learned to appreciate the process of learning.

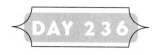

Jasmine and Dylan

To forgive myself for being a learner in this lifetime adds up when I think of how much I have learned and how it has benefited me. The pain, the suffering, the confusion, and the mistakes form a priceless education that has taught me exactly what I have needed to learn when I needed to learn it. This understanding deepens when I reflect on how my learning has benefited others. I ask myself if I would rather it had been my children, Jasmine and Dylan, surviving the abuse, the racism, the addiction, or whether I am content to have taken on the karma I have taken on so that they might not have to.

At some point our learning process becomes sacred to us and there is nothing to forgive.

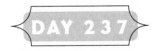

The Person and the Behavior

One of the pivotal insights I have gained as I practice self-forgiveness is an understanding of the difference between a person and a behavior. In the distorted world of greed, hatred, and delusion, two things that have nothing to do with each other often get treated as one. Freedom and violence, race and character, gender and ability come to mind when I think of this habit of the mind. Learning the skill of forgiveness, starting with ourselves, gives us our best chance of really understanding a person's frame of mind at the time of an unskillful behavior, our best chance to see how someone can feel as if they are doing the right thing or the best thing when they are coming from a confused and pained place.

This made a difference for me. I had thought forgiveness was about the behavior, but it's not; it's about the person. Whenever I meditated on a moment of my life, I could see through my younger eyes. I could feel what it was like to live with the confusion and pain that I was suffering from back then and see how the behavior did not need forgiveness; I did. We must forgive the person, learn from their behavior, and try to apply what we have learned.

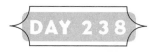

I Am Like That

Another insight I have gained from learning to forgive myself is that I am not so different from everybody else. As I learn about myself, a process that is impossible if we cannot forgive ourselves, I am learning about everyone else. I am getting to know what it is to be human. When I see another person in pain, behaving badly, I find myself softening and saying, "I am like that." That's what it's like being human sometimes, and being human is forgivable. When we forgive we get better, and when we get better what was dark and heavy becomes light.

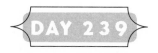

What Leads to the Heart

Ethical precepts and energy-raising practices move us out of the powerless place of the victim, empowering us to take ever-increasing responsibility for the choices that we make. The mindfulness practices of asana, *pranayama*, and meditation deepen both our capacity for and our commitment to conscious choice making. Our own suffering brings us, eventually, to the practice of compassion. All of these practices help us to understand the extent of human suffering in the world and inspire within us the desire to be of service. At this point we are small whirlwinds of potential energy seeking appropriate expression.

Loving-kindness is that expression.

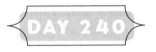

Loving-kindness

The practice of compassion has guided me into the posture of loving-kindness. Learning to forgive myself is teaching me to forgive everyone else and to see the people in my life as I am learning to see myself. As I go back into a moment of my life in which I was acting unskillfully, I can see one thing over and over again: love made a difference. The people in my life who were able to get past my defenses and were able to touch my heart were treasured.

When we are in suffering, love is like water in a desert. The longer I practice compassion, the more certain I am that no one is choosing suffering, yet there it is. I tell the teachers I train that we are the lucky ones. We have our practice and we have one another. When you go home tonight and into the world after this weekend, remember this and act accordingly; bring that water out into the desert, bring loving-kindness—all of us want to make a difference; start by bringing the most important thing.

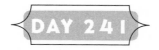

Metta, the Practice of Loving-kindness

Loving-kindness, or *metta* meditation, is the Buddha's response to the suffering he observed during mindfulness practice. The practice would later be validated by Western research into neuroplasticity, which has revealed that the brain creates associations between a smell and a moment in your life, a song and a relationship, a person and a feeling, the rule of thumb being "What fires together wires together." The Buddha created a practice that takes advantage of this habit of the brain: intentionally creating an association between the felt experience of loving-kindness and the people in our lives. We learn to associate the thought of a person with the heartfelt desire to offer loving-kindness. This learning process begins with us.

An intensely practical practice, in this kind of meditation the meditator patiently offers herself loving-kindness over and over again. After a while, she starts to do the same thing for a benefactor, then someone she feels neutral toward, and, finally, someone she finds difficult. Like forgiveness practice, we learn about why we should offer loving-kindness by offering it. While the brain is learning to associate this or that person with the act of offering loving-kindness, the mind is gathering insight into the process of transforming a relationship with a practiced intention. Like prayer, offering loving-kindness works. My students consistently report their relationships shifting toward kindness and connection as they practice the intention of kindness and connection.

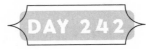

Safety, Health, Happiness, Community

The practice of offering loving-kindness is broken down into four categories: safety, health, happiness, and community. The phrases are: "May you be safe," "May you be healthy," "May you be happy," and "May you be at ease in your community," and they can be used during a ten-minute meditation or a three-month retreat. From those phrases a meditator or teacher can elaborate to her heart's content. I have found it easier to remember and easier to get some momentum built up when I keep it simple. I tend to hold a vision of what I am wishing for myself or someone else in my head as I repeat the phrases. I have also built these phrases into my life so that I am offering loving-kindness at the beginning and at the end of every class, workshop, or training I lead. Working these phrases into my everyday life has helped me to sustain my attention on the act of being kind and generous and how important it is to me. Most days the world's suffering appears unchanged by my practice; however, this is just a misunderstanding of my mind. The world and I only appear to be separate but we are as the ocean is to the wave. Every day that I practice loving-kindness, I change and the world changes with me. *Bhavantu.*

CHAPTER FIVE

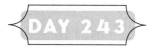

Moving Mountains

People tell me they shouldn't try yoga because they are not flexible, which is like saying we shouldn't go to the dentist because we have cavities. This is the way we often relate to the practices that will bring us back into balance. They tend to be the last thing we feel like doing. The habits that have taken us out of balance have a sort of negative holistic momentum that affects everything from our biochemistry to the friends we have chosen. Decades of this sort of momentum have a self-perpetuating logic of their own that is hard to argue with: "If you had my problems you would drink like this too"; "I would love to but who has the time?" This is where teachers, intentional spaces, and intentional communities step in to save us from ourselves.

The return to balance starts out of balance. To compensate for this we need people around us to guide our first steps and the willingness to take them. We begin the practice of loving-kindness meditation a country mile from balance. It is not in our nature to focus on the positive. Millions of years of evolution have taught us to stay alive by remembering the one snake in a meadow, relegating the flowers and sunshine to the portion of the brain that forgets. This works from a survival standpoint but it has turned our relationships into a running commentary on how things could be better.

Our first passes at offering ourselves loving-kindness often feel weak in the face of decades of self-criticism. We get that we need it, but is this going to be enough? The next day our teachers have us offer loving-kindness to ourselves and others again, the people around us quietly begin the process, and grudgingly we make a beginning and discover what our teachers discovered before us: that love is like water. One drop is not so powerful, a few more drops and things begin to change, enough drops and you can move mountains.

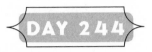

Starting with Ourselves

During my first years practicing loving-kindness meditation I found that offering loving-kindness to myself was a lukewarm affair, offering it to my benefactors was awesome, offering it to people I felt neutral toward was pleasant enough, and offering it to people I found difficult was, well, difficult. Being kind to a difficult person was preferable to being kind to myself because it was less boring, the way a horror movie, while not my first choice, is still less boring than a blank screen in an empty theater. My relationship with myself was somewhat more unsettling than my relationship with people I found difficult because at least with them I knew where I stood.

I call meditation practice a grown-up practice because it demands all of our resources and because it requires us to embrace a more mature perspective. Mindfulness practice made it possible to stay in the same posture long enough to see that I really wasn't engaged when it came to my relationship with myself. The weakness of my loving-kindness meditation was a reflection of the fact that I did not know who I was offering kindness to when I was offering it to myself. My teachers suggested that we stick with offering loving-kindness to ourselves until we felt ready to move on. I tried this and stuck with myself for a couple of years, slowly learning to face myself and to wish myself the best.

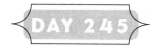

Learning to Be Kind

When I began this practice of loving-kindness, I was kind when it suited my conditioning, which is to say I had very little sway over when and where I would be kind and to whom. Although most of us have a pretty strong intention to be kind to those we love, we aren't all that interested in being kind to anyone else, and even our track record with those we love leaves a fair amount to be desired. Kindness is great, but we often have other priorities.

Holding the intention to be kind steadily over extended practice periods brings us in touch with all that competes with offering kindness: the self-absorption, the judgments, the fears, and the various states of distraction we fall into that turn us away from the simple, sacred task of being kind. When I think about being kind I think of my son, Dylan, who has been a perfect child, literally, his whole life. Kind, sweet, and funny, he has had a flawless report card since he began getting them and he doesn't even like school; he just knows his older sister gets straight As and assumes his family expects it of him. When we are together he is all smiles, laughter, love, and praise, and even with him I am still learning to choose kindness over the other ways I have learned to be.

CHAPTER FIVE

5

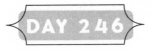

Our Benefactors

Offering loving-kindness to those who have helped us along the way is always a joy. At last, something to do on our meditation cushion that comes easily! It reminds us to be grateful and offers us something to aim at in our own lives: those who have helped us act as role models, demonstrating the many skillful attributes we hope to attain. Often these benefactors are no longer in our lives, and this meditation offers us a chance to give back to, make amends with, or gain closure with those we will never see again. It is a chance to honor those who helped us to get to this point, and commit to carrying the excellence they embodied forward.

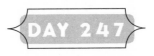

The Neutral Person

By the time we begin to offer loving-kindness to a person toward whom we feel neutral, we have already gotten a feel for the practice. It is something of a meditation field trip to remember someone you've seen that you have zero connection with and spend time wishing them the best. The practice begins with a review of your day. You reflect on the people you passed on the street or sat with on the bus, bringing awareness to any feelings you have for them, from attraction to aversion, and finding someone who is truly neutral. Holding this person in your mind's eye, you then spend a significant period of time offering them loving-kindness, connecting to the tenderness and generosity that your heart holds for everyone you meet.

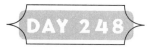

A Misunderstanding

The practice of yoga is the dissolving of a misunderstanding of the mind that begins and ends with the belief that we are separate from all that is, be it the natural world, our fellow human beings, or even ourselves. Time spent discovering our natural affection for people toward whom we consider ourselves neutral puts a significant dent in the assumption of separateness. The heart is drawn with compassion to the suffering we see in others and delighted by their happiness, and it holds a powerful generosity, wishing them all of the happiness we want for ourselves. While our heart is open to another person, our mind finds relief from the contracted states of greed, hatred, and delusion, returning effortlessly to spaciousness, ease, and clarity. Wanting the best for one another feels like sanity, salvation, and destiny. Wanting the best for one another feels like coming home.

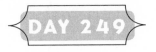

The Difficult Person

I didn't start holding grudges until late in life. During my years of active addiction I tended to run people over on my way to my next fix. This was never great for those involved, but it did have the advantage of being a short-lived affair. Sober, I had the bandwidth for long-term grievances. I had expectations, made assumptions, and when people failed to behave as expected or assumed, things got ugly. The suffering this newfound unskillfulness produced has been some of the most intense I have experienced in the last twenty years.

Enter the difficult person. To be clear, when we get to this person in our practice of loving-kindness, we are usually bringing to mind someone who has done actual, nontheoretical, heartbreakingly real harm to us. This is what makes them so difficult and why I needed to practice compassion formally before I could take this step in our practice. I needed to feel the legitimacy of separating the person from the behavior. Setting the behavior aside and offering kindness to the person has taught me four things:

1) It is possible to separate the person from the behavior in even the most challenging situations and have this separation make a difference to my heart and my mind.
2) What makes a person so difficult is the way they reflect the worst version of myself.
3) I, as an average person, have the ability to act beyond the "eye for an eye" paradigm. I can live with the responsibility to be kind in the absence of any "reason" to be kind. I can live with the possibility our greatest teachers have held out for us. I can live with love as my answer, no matter what.

4) If I hold anyone out of my heart, my heart will never be whole. This is why I have been so upset with the difficult person, because I feel as though they are making it impossible for me to succeed on my path. They are messing with my perfect world. What if my perfect world believes in me more than I believe in myself?

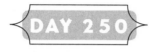

My Grandmother

My grandmother became pregnant with my mother and married my grandfather at the height of the Depression. This effectively closed most doors for both of them. They worked hard and provided for their three children. They lost loved ones in the wars that followed and gained more things too painful to talk about. My grandfather retired as a janitor with a pen from his boss and the emphysema he picked up at the factory. My grandmother made it to the typing pool before she retired. When my mom started adopting brown children, my grandfather seemed to get a kick out of it, but my grandmother burned with a rage that never cooled.

My experience of my grandmother was difficult. She seemed to actually hate me, but what was worse was the fear she put into my younger sister and the lack of respect she showed my older sister till the day she died. When I was young, my grandmother was just another potato in a really bad stew. As a sober adult, I felt she owed us more than she saw fit to give. I did not go to my grandmother's funeral and I did not go to her memorial service; I burned with a rage that never cooled. My practice has allowed me to see how each of us was protecting his or her heart from a world that felt too hard. I cannot forgive the abuse of children but I can understand a woman who felt utterly bereft of the life she wanted for herself. I can understand taking refuge in a rage that never cools, I can wish a young woman didn't have to, and I can know in my heart that if there were anything I could do to help I would.

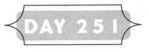

Mental Illness

My grandmother was an ordinary person contending with ordinary human suffering, but sometimes the people who do us wrong exhibit behaviors that are so beyond the pale—so devoid of empathy and compassion—that they are outside the realm of normal human behavior. Such people—murderers, rapists, and their ilk—are, in some way, disturbed and unwell. With my grandmother there was a person you could feel into. In other cases the person is buried deep under an impenetrable layer of illness. The method I was taught for offering loving-kindness is to find the person beneath the behavior, and in these cases, this often feels impossible. Because ordinary empathy is unavailable to them, the suffering this type of person can dish out is horrific. Practicing loving-kindness with these people is extremely difficult and should be done as a response to a genuine inner calling to do so from a safe physical, psychological, and emotional distance.

I have learned to give people the benefit of the doubt. If their behavior is beyond the scope of normality, then their suffering is as well.

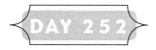

Wholeheartedness

Loving-kindness practice is like putting together a puzzle of a bridge over water. The sky parts are the benefactor, the earth on either side is the neutral person, I am the bridge, and the difficult person is the shadow beneath it. In each period of loving-kindness practice I find another part of the puzzle. On this day I find a bit of the sky, the next a bit of the bridge. Some days I find a lot, others are spent rummaging around wondering why I am doing this at all. As the puzzle fills in I am beginning to see that you could not have the bridge without the sky, the earth, and the shadow below. The many things are really one thing. The puzzle I am putting together is my heart and the image it portrays is my own true nature.

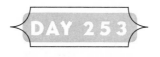

The Value of Compassion

It's as if we have our hand on a dial that determines the level of loneliness and isolation in our life. This dial also determines the amount of love and connection we have. The dial's name is compassion. What a blessing to know it exists. What an awakening to know that our hand is on this dial. How deep the urge to practice and to never forget once we have understood. How beautiful to share this understanding and this practice with others.

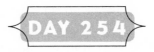

The Value of Kindness

The people I remember most are the ones who were kind to me when they did not need to be. The ordinary moments of kindness and generosity, the gentle word when I was in pain, the encouragement when I was doing my best. In those moments my faith in humanity and in myself was restored when I did not even know it had to be. This is the opportunity each of us has every moment of every day, to uplift another human being with just the smallest of gestures. No real cost, only kindness. It feels to me as if the fate of humanity rests in these moments. Will we take the time to be kind?

THREE WAYS TO PRACTICE COMPASSION AND LOVING-KINDNESS

1) Compassion: Sit quietly and review your life in ten-year increments, starting from when you were a child. Let a difficult or unskillful moment come to you. Feel how it felt to be in your body at that time. To see the world through your eyes as you were then. Then forgive yourself for being imperfect—for making mistakes—and for being a learner in this lifetime. Offer yourself forgiveness at least three times, then move to the next

decade of your life and repeat the process. Practice this as often as you need to, to become free.

2) Loving-kindness: The phrases are "May you be safe," "May you be healthy," "May you be happy," and "May you be at ease in your community." The practice is to spend time offering yourself these phrases, then a benefactor, then a neutral person, then a difficult one. When you are done, sit quietly for a while and feel into the energetic resonance of loving-kindness humming through your body and mind.

3) Use an abbreviated version of these practices and phrases throughout your day whenever you feel yourself contracting into negativity or expanding into the urge to pour love into the world.

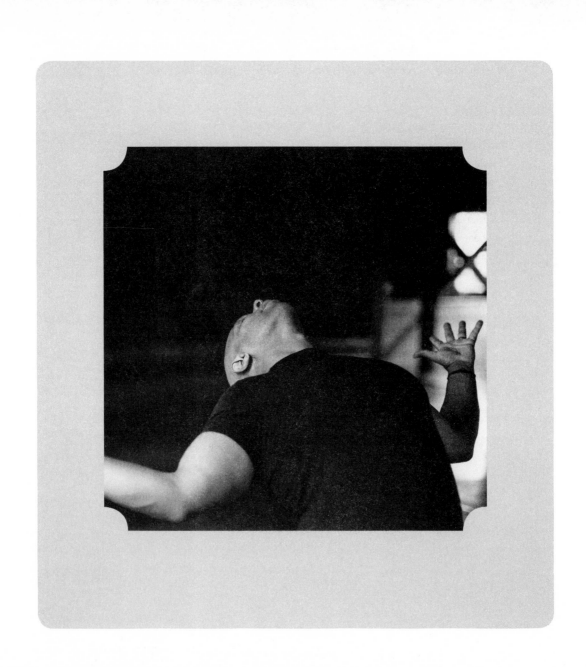

CHAPTER SIX

EQUANIMITY AND JOY

A child's life is full of promise and wonder because she has not yet contracted around this or that outcome, this or that narrative. As she moves into adulthood, she begins to specialize, becoming someone who does this and not that, someone who likes this and not that, someone who did this and not that. The story she creates about her life reflects the values of her time and place, her family and her community. Her world is measured from the outside in and contracts around this measurement. Her life is defined by her efforts to manage a contracted world that exists only in her mind. Then, one day, she goes to yoga and learns to reflect on her mind rather than to react from it.

The practice of mindfulness allows her to see the process of contraction in action as it unfolds from moment to moment. In time, she no longer needs to be taught about how greed, hatred, and delusion color her view; she can see it for herself. With a little more practice, she finds that she no longer takes the process personally; she accepts that it just is, like the weather. The habits of her mind that create suffering are like deer trails in a forest; if she does not use them, the forest will slowly erase them. Mindfulness allows her to patiently unlearn the trails she has contracted around and to create new ones that lead out of suffering.

Where once she lived within the narrow parameters of her conditioning, now she is feeling into the possibility of conscious choice making. Everything is now on the table. She busies herself cleaning up her inner and outer life, and one day, as she is putting her house in order, she finds something she did not know was lost. Resting in faded glory in the back corner of a forgotten cupboard is her heart. She spends an entire afternoon turning it over in her hands wondering what it means to have her heart back.

Compassion and loving-kindness are the first big adventures of her new life with a heart. She goes back to her old wounds and into her present passions with her eyes wide open and a renewed faith in herself and her world. It's dramatic and cathartic, romantic and turbulent. It is worthy of her and it would be enough. She moves into a place of authentic wholeheartedness. The people in her life recognize the worth she has brought into their own lives and what she does matters more than ever before. Her heart leads her down a new trail, a trail of accountability and service, a trail that teaches the paradox of generosity. She learns that she has to give it away to keep it.

Her life is full of promise and wonder, so full that her primary concern is no longer what she is receiving but what she is giving. She is learning to meet life's cycle of gain and loss, praise and blame, with equanimity. Content with the life she has chosen, the peace of her emotional maturity is sweetened by the joy she finds in the success of others as together they trudge the road to happy destiny.

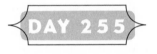

Two Definitions for Equanimity

There are two definitions of equanimity that form the basis of my practice. The first is not making a burden of our duties. This definition has gone a long way toward bringing the practice of equanimity into my daily life. The second is a steadiness or emotional unflappability through life's inevitable ups and downs. This definition has helped me with my erroneous expectation that life should be fair, as I define fair in the midst of a negative reaction to how things are going, and that has given me the ability to meet the unforeseen with clarity and calm, qualities those around me seem to prefer to confusion and chaos. In both cases, I am learning a new reaction to life—trust.

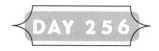

DAY 256

Three Reasons for Equanimity

The Buddha gives us three reasons to practice equanimity that stand the test of time. He tells us that we tend to think the impermanent is permanent, the unreliable is reliable, and that which is not the self is the self. He goes on to say that we get attached to our point of view and when life does not cooperate we suffer. The practices of mindfulness and compassion are tools for working with these habits of the mind. We experience an almost immediate shift in perspective from the beginning of our practice, and over time, we unlearn many of the habits of the mind that cause us to suffer. As this process takes place the tug of our old ways of seeing and being continue to cause suffering. The practice of equanimity allows us to be right there with the fact of our continued suffering, learning from it without taking it personally and seeing it for what it is: just passing through.

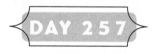

DAY 257

The Sun and the Moon

When I first came to meditation, my mindfulness levels were at rock bottom, but the thing that really got my goat was the injustice of how gain and loss, praise and blame, seemed to be handed out. It felt like my commitment

CHAPTER SIX

and effort were consistent, but the results just didn't add up. Life, it was clear to me, wasn't fair, and I could not let go of my reaction to this "fact."

A year or two into the process of sitting and breathing I realized I could live with life's not being fair, but I didn't have to like it. A couple of years later, I began to wonder why I was so self-centered. Things could have been a lot worse for me, and here I was complaining. Why did I have to see the glass as half-empty? Attacking my negativity seemed like taking the high road but it did not lessen my suffering. Mindfulness, compassion, and loving-kindness slowly arrested my negative inner dialogue and created a gentle space of watchfulness. I started to see the arising and passing of things differently. Everything was moving with a tremendous rhythm, blinking in and out of existence the way stars twinkle in the nighttime sky. Life, I realized, was actually sublime and had nothing to do with "fairness." Gain and loss, praise and blame, arise and pass like the sun and the moon moving through an eternal cycle. Watching as the world around me flowed into and out of existence, a question formed in my heart and mind together: "Which is better, the sun or the moon?"

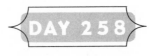

DAY 258

A Sun and a Moon

Lao-tzu wrote that the path forward seems to go back, and that the path into light seems dark. Often when you step onto the right path, it looks like you're taking a step backward toward the darkness of uncertainty. This has been my experience countless times in the last twenty-five years.

In 2004, I was driving the Massachusetts Turnpike in a brand-new car

CHAPTER SIX

going somewhere I had always wanted to go, doing something I felt I'd been born to do. In 2006, I was taking the train to New York City to be somewhere I did not want to be and to do something I did not want to do. On my way to Boston my eyes were closed to much of what I was a part of, and the ground underneath my feet did not belong to me. On my way to New York City my eyes were wide open and I was starting my life from the ground beneath my feet. I loved my time in Boston and it led to great suffering. I pretty much hated my time in New York and it led to self-respect and freedom. Which is better, the sun or the moon?

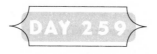

Not Making a Burden of Our Duties

In the world I grew up in, there was black and there was white, winners and losers, good and evil. In school, I divided my weeks into good and bad parts. The good part was the weekend and the bad part was the rest of the week. Fridays and Sundays were mostly good but they were unpleasantly tinged by their connection to the bad part of the week. I hated school and craved the end of it with my whole being. I counted days and died a thousand deaths. It was unmanageable.

My wife and I believe in public schools, the service they perform, and the ties our children have formed in our community by attending them. To align behind this value, I have had to apply yoga to the fact that my children and my entire family rhythm are now subject to a schedule that caused me so much suffering as a young person. I am teaching my children that it is not a problem to have duties and responsibilities. We all have them and they

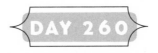

do not go away. We will be accountable to something till our last breath, so we might as well embrace it. My children have never known anything else and display courage and grace as they carry out the duties of being young. When they are afraid of something they are honest about it, and we work through it together, learning something valuable along the way. For my part, I am attempting to bring their example into the duties that make up the miracle that is my life.

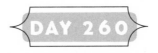

Locker Kit

My daughter is starting middle school tomorrow. I am in disbelief—and very proud. Last night, she showed me her locker kit. It is something her friends gave her to keep in her locker. She has filled it with everything a young person heading out on a new adventure needs. She talked me through each of the items and its uses: the hair ties, the spray-on dry shampoo, the hand cream. She's ready and she's excited. When I was a child I practiced fear; as an adult I am learning to practice equanimity. As I am learning to practice equanimity, my daughter is learning to practice the joy of living.

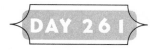

Resistance to the Pose Is Not the Pose

I often find myself teaching what it is I myself need to learn. My students remind me of how I am living and I teach them how being like me can be put to good use. In the hip-opening portion of my class there is a lot of shifting around and grimacing as people who have done intense cardiovascular exercise realize how stiff this has made their hips. They tend to keep shifting, never choosing a pose and working with it. There is the sense that this can't be right, and it is not. Shifting about is not the pose. Resistance to the pose is not the experience of the pose, it's just the experience of resistance. We need to become willing to start where we are, to commit to the pose, and to breathe into it.

Taking the train into New York City, to a place I did not want to be, to do something I did not want to do, I committed to the pose and began breathing into it. I began feeling into my life as it was and working with it. Within the space of only a couple of years I got to where I wanted to be and was doing exactly what I wanted to be doing. Showing up for a difficult duty taught me to acknowledge, to accept, and to understand. Showing up for a difficult duty taught me to live with humility, dignity, and equanimity.

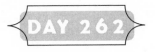

Making the Best of It

I ask the teachers I work with to practice making the best of things. To make the best of the training, to make the best of the opportunities they find in it, to make the best of me as a teacher, to make the best of the community we create together. I ask them to make the best of the training for their students and for themselves. I ask them to become accustomed to making the best of things because they will need to for the rest of their lives. They will go on to be leaders in their families and their communities, and those around them will depend on them to make the best of whatever the moment brings. To make the best of their skills, to make the best of their duties, to make the best of their relationships, to make the best of their precious human life. This is the yoga they will teach and there is no other.

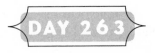

Learning to Bloom Where We Are Planted

For a while I felt like luck and circumstance decided success, but I have learned that success is really the ability to bloom where you are planted. Once this became clear to me I was able to see how whatever the moment brought was either something I was going to use to create success or something I was going to use as an excuse for not doing so. In either case, I was going to be the deciding factor, not my circumstances. Equanimity is the embodied expression of this understanding.

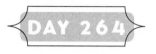

Control

As far as I can tell I have not been particularly greedy, hateful, or delusional when it comes to material things. I come from a family with four children, and the money we had was stretched pretty thin. I just never developed a sense that I needed a lot of things to be happy. Where my greed shows up is in my desire for control. My hatred is reserved for things that make me feel powerless, and I am delusional concerning most things related to control, the degree to which it is possible, and the benefits that can be derived from it. What I want to control is "my life," which is to say, my experience. Drugs and alcohol gave me the ability to choose my experience with enough certainty that I became addicted to them. The aspects of yoga that offered an immediate effect gave me the sort of control that I was looking for and—to some extent—obscured my practice's true benefits for a while. Significant life consequences forced me to get honest about this aspect of my relationship to yoga. Using yoga to "take the edge off" is better than using Valium, but it is not going to effect the positive change yoga represents. My practice can be an aspect of what has kept me stuck or it can be an aspect of what sets me free. It's my call.

Control flows from attachment to what we like and aversion to what we do not like. The desire for control turns plain old-fashioned wanting and not wanting into an ethos, a grand design, a sociopolitical theory, the hardened shell of a false self. I think of this trap as a big hole that we dig for ourselves and then fall into so that all we can see are the walls of our mind-made prison. This book is to a large extent an outgrowth of my experience climbing out of that hole and the adventures I have had embracing life on life's terms. Praise and blame are powerful felt experiences that trigger my desire for control, yet they have also provided me with a perfect space in which to practice letting go.

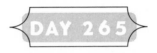

Praise and Blame

As a child in America, I was labeled a "Negro," a term that suggested a great deal of implicit blame. "Negro" men were dangerous, violent outlaws, and they didn't belong anywhere I tended to go. Nice people weren't "Negros." The white kids I met would look me over and then try to get back to what they were doing, their day somewhat disturbed by the implications of a "Negro" showing up. To make matters worse, I was an energetic male, which would be appreciated once I joined the workforce, but when I was a child it tended to attract a lot of negative attention. I learned to hate the experience of blame.

Black men were making a name for themselves in sports and I saw myself as being cut from their cloth. As an adolescent I found sports teams to be a place where I could belong and earn praise. I worked for years to become a wrestling champion, and on a March day, a ref raised my hand; I had done it. There is a picture of my mother hugging me after a particularly hard-fought victory, and it is the moment of purest love that I have ever experienced with her. I learned to crave the experience of praise. There have been times since when I have been upset with myself because it has taken me so long to develop equanimity about the way I am perceived by those around me, times when I could not forgive myself for being a learner in this lifetime. These days, I meet those moments with a compassion that softens into equanimity.

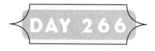

Standing in Welcome

To live with equanimity is to develop an inner life that is independent of whatever circumstances we find ourselves in. What grants us our freedom is not a devaluing of the world around us, it is the understanding that we are not our thoughts. The practice of mindfulness is the first step in this process, teaching us to reflect on the mind rather than to react from it. In time we come to see the space around our thoughts as being more important than our thoughts themselves, and we learn to rest in that space. The practices of the heart teach us that standing in this space with kindness and compassion is the true practice of yoga, and to let go of the rest. What follows is the ability to welcome whatever the moment brings.

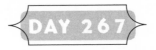

Forest Pool

My teachers have shared with me the image of a forest pool resting in stillness and the wondrous creatures that come to drink from its waters. How that pool welcomes all creatures equally, delighting in the unique qualities of each, and how they come to share themselves with the pool. My first take on this image was that it felt preposterously monastic and checked-out. Yeah, right, like I welcome a day at the beach, the IRS, Christmas morning, and diarrhea with equal delight. This reaction to the forest-pool image flowed from my mistaken belief that life was supposed to do what it was told and if it did not it was being bad.

My practice has taught me to enjoy life as an ongoing co-creative act. It began with teaching yoga. I could go to class, but the class did not happen until I interacted with whoever showed up. On my mat, I learned to flow with my limitations when it came to time or injury and learned to see how each new limitation brought with it a new possibility. On my cushion things took longer because I somehow found it possible to take things more personally than I had on my mat or while teaching. Eventually I found the forest pool deep within me, deep within the moment. Having abandoned time and judgment, my practice has become a possibility that does not happen until wondrous creatures arrive; I await them with equanimity and receive them with an active interest. I guess the delight comes later.

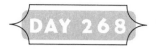

What the Wondrous Creatures Have to Say

Like most people, I tend to react to things that contradict my own story about myself. If someone says to me, "I like what you like," I can roll with it. The same is not true when my story is not validated. When I hear, "I do not agree with your ideas," I am prone to interpret the message as "I do not agree with your existence." Reflecting on rather than reacting to the wondrous creatures that come to drink at my pool is teaching me that I think something, then it becomes my idea, and once it becomes my idea, it becomes me. True, this makes no sense, but think about what happens when someone drives by with a bumper sticker that does not agree with one of your ideas, or a family member chooses not to validate your point of view. Worse yet, think about what happens if the bumper sticker or family member mocks one of your beliefs. Feel your reaction in the body, the breath, and the mind and see if you and your ideas have not become one and the same. The wondrous creatures that come to my pool are politely telling me to watch my mind and meet what I find there with compassion and equanimity.

DAY 269

Blame

When I am on the receiving end of blame, my physical body, my emotional body, and my mental body go on red alert. At this point I will usually either attack those blaming me or attack myself for putting me in a position to be blamed. This is true for blame that I feel is aimed at me personally and for blame that is aimed at things that I identify with. As a yoga teacher, when people say negative things about yoga, I react in much the same way as if they had said negative things about me personally. When my "side" wins, I win; when it loses, I lose.

My reaction to blame is a double whammy. The reaction itself is one form of suffering: I feel fear, anger, and confusion, with a side of guilt and shame—if for no other reason than that I resent myself for landing in these sorts of situations. In addition to the suffering brought on by my reaction, there is also the suffering of confusion this reaction creates. Clear seeing and contracted states cannot coexist. I find myself in need of an appropriate response while trapped in a reaction that makes that response next to impossible. This is why I set aside time each day to practice reflecting and not reacting. Through yoga we learn to reflect on and not react to the fact that we are in a state of reaction. When the wondrous creature of blame arrives and our mind-body reacts, there will be a part of us that is grounded, observant, and able to choose wisely no matter what.

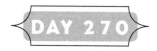

Being Right or Being Wise

I was taught that there are no straight lines in nature. That straight lines only exist in our mind. One of the straight lines our mind tries to draw is the one that connects our thoughts and our actions to being right. It is one of our most cherished delusions that we are right all the time. We are so attached to this delusion that we react strongly to anything that threatens it. But often what we are rejecting is the very information we need in order to find happiness. The irony of this situation is not lost on anyone who has ever tried to help another human being. The practice of yoga is a safeguard against the habit of the mind to see only what it wants to see. What I am finding is that this sort of suffering reminds me that I can be right or I can be happy, that I can be right or I can be wise.

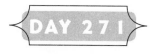

Taking Responsibility

The tenth step in the twelve-step program tells us that when we are wrong we should admit it promptly. It's a great habit to embrace for several reasons. People tend to trust us more when they know that we will admit when we are wrong. When we can be honest, problems are addressed as an acorn and not an oak tree. I learned this practice as a young person and

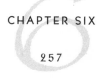

immediately felt the difference between taking responsibility and accepting blame. Accepting blame felt like accepting shame. Taking responsibility felt like accepting my true power in a situation. Accepting blame perpetuated a negative narrative. Taking responsibility transformed a negative situation into a positive one. Accepting blame happened from the outside in. Taking responsibility happened from the inside out. Taking responsibility for my actions, although sometimes uncomfortable, was powerful evidence that I had left the life of the addict and victim behind and was choosing to live according to spiritual principles. Accepting blame was something I did with my head held low. Taking responsibility was something I learned to do with my head held no higher and no lower than anyone else's.

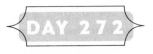

The Calm Part

Today was the first day back at school for my two children. My daughter tends to be excited and optimistic. My son, Dylan, tends not to think about it until the morning arrives, then gets butterflies. I was meditating before we left and heard my wife ask Dylan if he was anxious. "No, Mom, I am not anxious; I'm scared," he replied. I called him in to where I was sitting and had him meditate with me. He has always been a skilled meditator; he can meditate so deeply that he is immune to tickling.

When we were done I asked him if he'd been able to move into his body and his breath and find calm there. He said he had. I told him that the calm is always there. There is the scared part of you, mostly in the mind, and there is the calm part of you, in your body and your breathing. The scared part is just there to remind you of the calm part. I told Dylan that yoga is first learning to move into the calm part when we are caught up in a lot of negative feelings. And then it is learning to be with our feelings from the calm part.

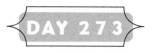

Praise

Offering heartfelt praise to someone who is embodying an ideal that we aspire to is a powerful way of connecting to our own highest aspirations while affirming our connection with, and appreciation for, another human being. Manipulative praise, while self-destructive for the person offering it, has the merit of forcing the would-be manipulator to acknowledge the presence of virtue. The real danger of praise is both that it has the potential to give us an inaccurate sense of who we are and that we can become attached to it.

Because praise is something I learned to covet at an early age, my seeking it became so ingrained in me that for a long time it was a largely unexamined force in my life. Like alcohol, it was something I always wanted more of. Sitting and breathing, I have discovered that there are entire parts of my life that have been labeled that way: either "all good" or "all bad." Praise has seemed "all good," most of my life, without a moment's reflection. It was only after beginning yoga that I began to ask, "Why is praise good? What amount of praise do I need? What do I need praise for?"

I now see praise as an aspect of healthy mirroring like healthy eating. Like food, praise of the right kind and in the right amounts is powerful medicine. When I praise my children, my wife, my friends, and my students for a job well done I see them glow in the light of love like a plant in the light of the sun. Skillful praise is a way for us to affirm one another as we perform the hard work of a good life.

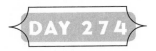

See, Meet, Respond

One of the challenges of teaching teachers is giving them something they can remember, use easily under pressure, and teach to students who will in turn also have to remember it under pressure and apply it to the choices they make. Taking a teaching like the first chapter of the Yoga Sutras and boiling it down to a skillful way of being that someone I will never meet can practice at work and at home has taken some time. The following formula is what I've come up with: I believe the first chapter of the Yoga Sutras is teaching us to see clearly, meet what we see with compassion, and then respond with kindness. Seeing, meeting, and responding are to be practiced with joy and equanimity.

There is a time for seeing praise for what it is, then meeting our own relationship to praise and the person offering it with compassion and responding to them with kindness.

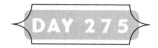

Winning and Losing

At times, my love of praise has come at the expense of my indifference to the costs others have had to pay in order for me to be a winner. I did not invent this indifference; it has been practiced by humanity for as long as there have been winners and losers. But I am responsible for how *my* behavior affects others. To practice equanimity around praise I have had to learn three things:

1) Things change.
2) The easiest way for me to perpetuate suffering in my life is to become attached to outcomes and to define my identity by them.
3) I live an interdependent life. When I receive praise, the countless others who helped make what I do possible receive it as well.

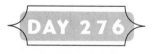

Gain and Loss

Due to a lawsuit with a business partner, I had to sell the house I had grown up in because I could no longer afford it. Today other people's children play on the lawn my parents had hoped to watch their grandchildren run across. When I sold my first book I was able to afford a high-definition television and a DVD player to go with it. The pride and happiness I felt watching movies on that television with my wife on summer evenings is something I will never forget.

When my friend Jude died it meant I would never see him again. Ever. Everything we had ever done together will forever belong to the story of someone who died alone and before his time. When I remember his laugh, I remember how he died. Life is filled with gain and loss. What remains to be seen is how we will learn to live with what has been gained and what has been lost.

The fact that the reactions we form in response to gain and loss are grounded in actual events does not change the facts of suffering and the end of suffering. The fact that these gains and losses are real does not change the fact that when we believe the impermanent is permanent, the unreliable is reliable, and that which is not the self is the self, we suffer.

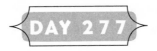

Impermanence

The first thirty-five years of my life were spent without any awareness that impermanence was something I should even be thinking about, let alone meditating on. Things came and went; so what? Indeed.

Impermanence itself is not the problem—in fact we could fill volumes with the things we are glad are impermanent. We could start with wars. I am particularly glad when impermanence brings me the things I like. Spring in the wake of a New England winter is an excellent example. The same is also true when impermanence takes away things I don't like; poison oak is presently receding from my left arm due to impermanence, and I am thankful for it. Impermanence keeps things interesting and makes life possible; we could not breathe if the inhale did not give way to the exhale.

Suffering happens when we do not see the impermanent for what it is. My teachers kept it simple; they taught me that we should watch the arising and passing of things. That we should just watch; that we should be right there as the in-breath ends, that we should be right there as the out-breath ends, that we should be right there as the sound of the bell vanishes into silence. They taught me that we should learn to appreciate the ubiquitous nature of impermanence and to appreciate each moment as it dances onto the stage of life, takes a bow, and dances off again.

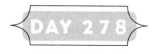

Fearlessness

As my investigation into the nature of impermanence began to mature, I found a new gear. Up to that point in my practice I'd had an average amount of nostalgia and attachment toward things that came and went. I suffered, as most of us do, when things I had grown to appreciate or love vanished and things I was unsure of arose. I do not think I was exceptional in any sense; I just think I was experiencing ordinary suffering. Sitting and breathing, I began to appreciate the rhythm of things, the rhythm of my own experience. I found that I could love the sound of the bell as it arose. As the sound of the bell lasted I found I could love that too. And as the sound of the bell vanished, I could love that as well. It was no longer appropriate for me to live in fear of life's true nature. As people, places, and things danced into and out of my life, I began to practice living in fear less, offering each moment its due.

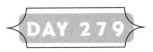

Max

The week after I became a yoga teacher I adopted a six-month-old puppy. My wife and I named her Max and she shared our lives for fourteen years. Max possessed a full measure of all the things that make dogs awesome. There was a twinkle in her eye, a spring in her step, and wherever her loved ones could be found, that was her home. She treated loving my wife and me as her full-time job and I loved her back with every cell in my body. When I was walking to work she was at my side. When I ran groups with children she was under the table. When I taught yoga she waited for me in the teachers' room. When I hiked the mountains of Western Massachusetts she was scouting ahead. When I brought my two children home from the hospital she met them with a smile. She was with me for the first fourteen years of my life as a yoga teacher and I could not have succeeded without her. Then, one morning, she was through. There was no fear, and whatever pain she was in did not reach her eyes. She was just a little embarrassed that she could not do her job anymore. I took her to the vet and held her in my arms as she died. She gave me a great life and I gave her the best death I could.

Life will teach us to love and to let go whether we want it to or not.

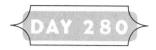

Unreliability

To better understand this next form of suffering we might consider the experience of owning a car. The car comes and goes, and while we are in possession of it, it changes, from new to old. The coming and going is impermanence. The depreciation of the car is unreliability. Things do not need to vanish in order to change their nature. The car that is shiny and new and brings us pleasure becomes the car that is old and rusty and causes us embarrassment.

The practice of mindfulness brings us right there for the arising and passing of the moment. A refinement of that process is to watch how even the objects that do not vanish are in a constant state of transformation. When I was young, I appreciated the effect this process had on my jeans, slowly fading them to just the right color. But I did not appreciate the fact that it also blew out the knees, making them useless. We want our ducks to get in a row, but in doing so we miss the point of living. Impermanence got our ducks in a row and impermanence will get them out of a row. It's all the same thing. The world that brings us everything we need for this human adventure we call life does so by remaining in a constant state of transformation. What we call unreliability is actually the process of creation itself.

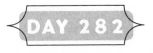

Creation

Deepak Chopra teaches us that when we hold an intention, it organizes its own fulfillment. That our intention acts on the field of pure potentiality and organizes an infinity of time-space events. The fabric of the universe unravels and re-forms around our heart's desires, and when that process is over it begins again, the form of our old life fading and eventually vanishing in order to create the form of our new one. Yoga would have us be right there for everything, without getting lost in or dishonoring the moment by thinking that what we are watching is anything other than what it is, the miracle of creation. The world around us—the trees, the rocks, the oceans—participate in this miracle without understanding it. Without the ability to know it for what it is. That is our job.

DAY 282

Seeing

If we could speed up how we see, the way they do with time-lapse photography, we would find that the world around us is in a state of constant transformation, organizing for a moment to express one of an infinity of truths, then dissolving to form the next.

We cannot change the way we see. We cannot slow down or speed up the way our eyes take in light, so we must learn to change the way we use our ability to see, instead. Before meditation, when I saw something, I drew on my past experiences to understand it, until I felt confident that I "knew" what it was. This was now my chair, my parking spot, my space in the yoga studio. I was using my "self" and my experience to measure the world. Yoga has taught me to see the world differently, by showing me a different way to measure it.

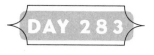

A World That Vanishes

Would courage exist if we did not live in a world that vanishes? Would inspiration exist if we did not live in a world that vanishes? Would there be anything to say in a world that did not vanish? Would children ever grow to make their parents' hearts burst with pride and love if we did not live in a world that vanishes? Would we be able to meet our death in the manner in which we met our life in a world that did not vanish? Would there be victory or the end of a worthy task done with great love if we did not live in a world that vanishes? Would we cheer for athletes, artists, musicians, writers, actors, teachers, and those who give their lives in the service of their communities if we did not live in a world that vanishes? Could we love as deeply as we do if we did not live in a world that vanishes?

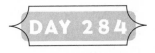

Under a Nighttime Sky

I was living in New York when I started attending retreats at Spirit Rock Meditation Center in Northern California. My first roommate there had grown up and still lives in San Francisco. The last night of our first retreat together we talked into the wee hours about his life in the Bay Area and his experience as a member of the Spirit Rock community. Over the years we have often found ourselves attending the same retreats and have fallen into a tradition of walking out under the stars on the last night to find a bench and tell each other how our lives have changed since we last met. We are both self-employed fathers and share many of the same joys and concerns. Nothing ever happens the way we thought it would and everything is always better than we could have hoped. There have been times of great difficulty and times of great good fortune for both of us. We have needed to make difficult choices and practice principles that were not obviously in our best interest. We have not been immune to praise and blame, gain and loss, but we share the practice of mindfulness and compassion, and that has been more than enough.

Leaving the bench, walking back to our dorms, the life we have lived begins to fade and the life we will live starts to form. Together we stop to take in a deep breath under the nighttime sky.

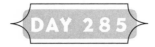

DAY 285

Mom and Dad

In my experience the family connections created by adoption are different from the family connections formed by genetics. My children and I share a world in common: our eyes, our hands, our feet, our skin, our sense of humor, and the rhythm of our minds. Each of us expresses a different aspect of the same theme. This sameness creates an effortless bond. When we are together nothing is lacking.

The family my mom and dad put together was more like a car made from spare parts. Each of their adopted children was emerging from the experience of utter abandonment, and my parents had lost three biological children before deciding to adopt. We were a family of the bereft. It was hard and often tragic. My mom and dad kept working at being parents and I kept working at being their son. As the years have passed, the distance between us, the wounds, the wrongs, the reasons not to forgive, have all faded. Our reasons not to love one another were unreliable. The ways that we have fallen short and were less than we could have been turned out to be unreliable as well. As my mom and dad come to the end of their lives, they know that they have been able to love with all their hearts, which is proving to be the most reliable measure of a good life. They are content and so are their children.

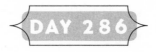

That Which Is Not the Self

The Yoga Sutras teach that we get things mixed up. We think we are the car we own or the job that we have. When things are going well with the car or the job we experience joy and equanimity; when things get tough at work or the car breaks down, our inner life changes like the surface of a lake reflecting clouds moving across an afternoon sky. We think it is normal to believe that we are separate from the world around us and to be completely at its mercy at the same time. This is the impossible situation that yoga is trying to help us resolve. First, we notice that we, and the world we are a part of, are in a constant state of transformation and that our mind tends to find fault with this. After a period of reflection on the body, the breath, and the moment we are ready to look at what is and what is not the self. Hint: we are looking for what is looking.

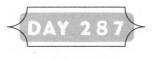

Yoga

Looking back on them, my first experiences of yoga have a comic quality. Pretty much everything that I was taught I had never heard of, or thought of, before, and the assumptions that I made were often preposterous. The word "mindfulness" sounded like something I would get around to if I had no life, "compassion" was for hypocrites who were hiding out from their anger, and "awareness" seemed both mundane and to require some sort of special ability that I lacked. Because of the assumptions I made about myself, the world I was living in, and the people I was interacting with, I simply could not imagine that what I was being taught was relevant to me in any meaningful way.

Nearly twenty years later, I have a sense of what my teachers meant by "awareness," and how mindfulness is the study of our participation in it. That there is the brain and then there is the mind, which is what the brain is doing. The experience of the mind is consciousness, which has the capacity to bring the individual and the universal perspectives together and to enact this union, this yoga, within what we call the here and now.

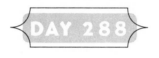

Finding Myself

It is one thing to read about an experience—like watching your daughter come into the world—or to be comforted by the experiences of those who have gone before us on a path. To be guided by them as we move toward our own authentic choices. It is quite another thing to live the breathtaking moments of direct experience, when a dream is being realized. The moment when we are gliding across the surface of the water on a surfboard for the first time; the moment standing at the altar when your bride appears around the corner, her father by her side, the dress, the smile.

A couple of years ago I spent a week at a retreat in which the only guidance was to "be right there at the beginning of the in-breath," morning, noon, and night. Far into this retreat, long after I had any hope of ever doing anything else for the rest of my life, something different happened. I came to this particular practice period with no expectations I just took my seat and got set. Phillip Moffitt was teaching that morning, and after a period of settling in, he asked us to move our attention from the breath to the space of the room around us and to the quality of pure knowing that is taking in that space. I did. He asked us if there was a self in the space and sounds of the room. There was not. He then asked if there was a self in the sensations of the body and the breath. There was not. I was as present as I had ever been in my life and there was no self to be found anywhere, just sensations—pure knowing—and the experience of knowing that I was knowing.

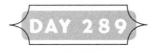

Ducks

My wife says that the more I meditate the more I laugh, and I have to agree with her. Part of it is an expression of compassion, kindness, equanimity, and joy. People are full of fear and suffering, and laughing makes us feel better. Laughing often and easily soothes our suffering, and the suffering of those around us.

I also laugh because the practice of mindfulness reveals ordinary life to be exactly like the Bill Murray movie *Groundhog Day*, only in this version we never learn. Jill won't talk to Jane because she didn't do what Jill thinks she would have done in Jane's place. Bill wants Bob to do this but it is the last thing that Bob will do, just because Bill wants him to. Keeping score and holding grudges like a boss, caught in the trap of measuring the world by our own standards and wanting everyone to agree with us. If our interpersonal relationships weren't challenging enough there's the ducks to think about. Every time we get our ducks in a row they wander off and we get bent out of shape, rather than looking at why we think a row of ducks matters so much. It's as if we are afraid of what life would be like if we weren't so unhappy. Preferring an unhappiness that is false to a happiness that is real, we make a stranger of the truth.

I laugh because we know better; if we didn't it wouldn't be funny.

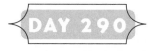

Empty of That

My teachers shared with me a story about the Buddha meeting with a student. To help the student understand the concept of emptiness, he asked the student if he was familiar with the town that surrounded the park where they were meeting—the people selling things, the sounds, the smells, the wealth, the poverty, the busyness. The student said he was familiar with all of these things. Then the Buddha said, "This park is empty of that." Once I got sober my life became empty of active alcohol addiction. Once I began forgiving myself, my life began to become empty of the judgment and the self-righteousness it once held. The practice of mindfulness is teaching me to become empty of the notion that I can find myself in the impermanent and the unreliable. With each year of practice I am a little emptier in general. This might sound like a bad thing, but it is quite the opposite. Being empty feels like coming home, being grounded and at ease. Being empty allows love and inspiration to move through me like a breeze through a night-time sky. Being empty is allowing this book to write itself. Being empty is effortless. When I am empty I can be right there for the felt experience of this body, this breath, this moment, without commentary. Attachment closes all of this off like a knot in a water hose. Yoga is giving me the chance to become empty of that.

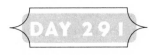

DAY 291

This Business of Winning and Losing

I was sitting in a twelve-step meeting as the first Iraq war was winding down and a woman next to me commented that we appeared to have won. As she considered this she said she was no longer clear about this business of winning and losing anymore. It was one of those moments when you feel like you are waking up from a dream. Sitting at a twelve-step meeting in a church basement, I was being given permission to become empty of a misunderstanding I had held all my life: the misunderstanding of trying to find myself in a world divided into "winning" and "losing."

I realized that I was clinging to this false dichotomy out of habit and a sense that there was no alternative. I did not stop clinging to those beliefs that day, but my grip began to loosen and my mind began to open. My life was becoming empty of winning and losing. It was a perfect first step. In the years since, my life has become empty of other misunderstandings, many of them rooted in a mistaken belief that I "should" be something that I am not.

Each time I become empty of another fiction I do not go anywhere, I do not become less, I just stand in the world a little easier. Each time I become empty of a fiction, I am making room for the truth.

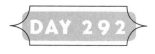

Thirst

It's important to be still and watch. Within the space of ten to fifteen minutes you will see everything. There will be pleasant things you want to stay that leave. There will be unpleasant things you want to leave that are only made worse by your wanting them to go. There will be neutral comfort zones that you will become attached to without even knowing they were there until they leave. You will find that everything that moves through your awareness comes and goes—nothing stays except awareness itself. While it's there the sensation, the thought, the desire, the aversion changes. The pain deepens, then shifts to another part of the body. The grudge runs hot, then becomes exasperation at having to go back over the same old ground.

Even you change. In the space of ten or fifteen minutes you are ten to fifteen people. The person winning at meditating, the person losing at meditating, the person who is blessed to be meditating, the person who is cursed to be meditating, the angry person, the bored person, the person who won't peek at her watch, the person peeking at her watch.

All of this is miraculous. Within us is a universe that is in a state of constant transformation. Watching our inner life, we can become more attuned to the patterns and rhythms of the natural world around us and to the inner

CHAPTER SIX

lives of the people we share it with. Or we can thirst for the pleasant to stay and the unpleasant to go so intensely that we confuse the experience of life with the experience of our thirst. Having arrived at this misunderstanding we can defend it to the death, clinging to a way of being that is causing us to suffer. Yoga offers those of us who can no longer tell the difference between living and thirsting a chance to become empty of that.

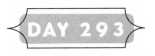

Win-Win

Equanimity is a watershed state of consciousness. It is the moment when we have found our balance in life. We have learned to surf the waves of praise and blame, gain and loss, and are content to play the hand life is dealing us. Having changed the way we are seeing and being, the world as we see it changes. The sorrows and joys of others affect us differently. The work we are doing with compassion and loving-kindness has taught us to see the person behind the behavior. As we have learned to forgive ourselves we have become less blinded by judgment in our relationships. Empathy is a skill we can now be counted upon to bring to whatever challenges our loved ones or communities are facing. We can finally understand that when those around us win, we win, and that it is the only way we have ever won.

CHAPTER SIX

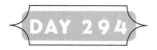

Joy

The first truly sane state of mind I ever moved into with any regularity was gratitude. As a newly sober young person I could reflect on the miracle of my sobriety and experience an upwelling of love, peace, and purpose whose name was gratitude. Taking my seat at a twelve-step meeting, sitting on the subway on my way to work, walking down the street in a body that had not been poisoned the night before, with an inner life that was not awash with guilt and shame, I was never far from breaking into eye-watering gratitude. To this day, my experience of gratitude has an effect like grief washing over me, taking my breath away, forcing me to put down everything else and bear witness to it. They say a grateful heart will never drink; I say a grateful heart will never do harm and will gladly give its last beat in the service of others. There was a long period during which gratitude was the only feeling I could trust, and I have dedicated my adult life to expressing that feeling.

The practice of yoga taught me to feel into the experience of safety, contentment, peace, love, affection, kindness, self-respect, purpose, determination, flow, and, above all, humor. These feelings have filled my life as I have progressively become empty of fear and anger. Fear and anger are dense states, crowding out everything else. Skillful states, like flow and ease, are empty and afford plenty of room for emotional range and nuance. Equanimity, in particular, sets the stage for a state of mind that I now put on the same level as gratitude. The joy we can find in others' success is a particularly powerful state of mind. Like gratitude, it has the ability to transport us out of whatever contracted state we are stuck in and into the bliss of being.

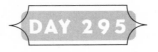

Having Heroes

It helps to have heroes. People whose lives bring a smile to our faces, people who teach us how to live by how they live. Giving our attention to the greatness we see in another person awakens that same quality in us. We get confused because our own greatness will never look like theirs, but it is there nonetheless. We have so much value and virtue within us that we need assistance finding it, naming it, choosing it. Our heroes help us with this, offering their lives as a measure, giving shape to things, pointing us in the right direction. Preparing us for the moment when life turns to us with both joy and sadness in her eyes, to say, "You're up."

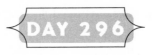

The Next Generation

The final chapter of the Yoga Sutras breaks life into four parts: we discover our gifts, develop them, learn to enjoy them, and then learn to let go. The third aim of life—that we learn to enjoy it—is one of sustainability. It's when we learn to put together not days or years but decades. The only way we can put three, four, five decades of contented service together is by thinking of the next generation, thinking about their challenges, their opportunities, their burdens, and their happiness. In the first two aims of life

CHAPTER SIX

278

we are developing our gifts and offering them to those around us. With the third we are learning to share them with people we will never meet as they face challenges we will not live to see.

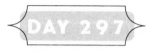

Passing It On

When I needed to get sober there was a seat waiting for me in twelve-step meetings all over the world. When I needed to heal there were yoga mats and meditation cushions waiting for me everywhere I went. When I needed to learn about life I found instructions that countless generations had dedicated their lives to passing on. A torch of wisdom and compassion passed down from generation to generation through the light and shadow of human history. I fell in love with the process of conveying the message of yoga and became a teacher. This was easier said than done. I have found myself brought to my knees and sometimes laid flat on my back. Like a boxer using the ropes to get back up, I have found my way to my feet not with a vision of what I could *get* but what I could *give*. There is tremendous power and joy in taking responsibility for passing on what has been given to us, in saying thank you to the countless individuals you never met by attempting to help countless others that you will never know.

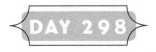

Using My Eyes

I tell the teachers I train to use their eyes. "Look at your students and use the skills and principles of yoga to build a class around what you see." This is challenging because they have to create the class as it happens instead of simply imposing their will or a plan on a class. It's harder, but it works better. I taught this initially as a practical skill: teach to what is happening in the room. Over time, I have come to see a deeper dimension to this style of teaching. If I use my eyes I have to develop my teaching style around the changing needs of my students. As the students grow and change, my teaching grows and changes too. My teaching cannot grow and change unless I do. If I use my eyes I will grow and change as my students do.

The possibility that a teacher could grow and change as her students do speaks to a deeper dimension of the practice of joy. On the surface of it, practicing joy is a practical response to the fact that your odds of finding happiness go way up if you can find it not just in your own good fortune but in the good fortune of everyone. You are casting a way wider happiness net.

The practice of joy also serves to connect us intimately with the lives of others. As our hearts and minds open in joy at how others are succeeding, we become available to the true diversity of human achievement. In joy, we feel into potentialities and possibilities within ourselves that we could never have imagined had we not understood them and affirmed them in others.

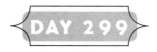

Joy as Mindfulness

Joy dials us into the world around us. Our attention is right there, our hearts are open, our minds are open, and our motivation is to know what is true. We are standing in compassion, with an attitude of loving-kindness, and the joy that we feel is without attachment, nothing extra. Caring deeply with an open heart and an open mind, we have the felt experience of the world around us. I was in Germany when the Berlin Wall came down. The following summer Germany won the World Cup, and I definitely felt a lot of the joy that the German people were feeling. It felt like the grass and the trees were happy. It felt like their nightmare was finally coming to an end and that a new future was available to them. There was no self in this understanding of the world around me, just empathy, appreciation, and joy. In this selfless connection, my understanding of falling down and getting up was forever changed.

The applications of this kind of mindfulness are infinite. I have learned to be a teacher, a parent, a husband, and a friend practicing the mindfulness that joy creates. Joy puts us right there with an open heart and an open mind, learning what we need to learn in an effortless space of love and appreciation.

CHAPTER SIX

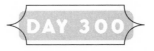

The Edge of My Seat

To train a teacher you must let them teach. To get them ready for this there is a period in each training that is the "Rolf Gates Show," in which I give the talks and teach the classes. If I do my job right this is over and done with before we are halfway through. As soon as possible I move to the back of the room and the students start giving the talks and leading the classes. I love this part of training because it is so completely efficient. The student will never look at the material as intently as she does when she's getting ready to teach it to her peers. Her experience of actually delivering a talk or a class is 100 percent preparation for doing so in the real world. Her perspective on the material adds a dimension to the training that would not be possible without her efforts. The rest of the students get to see a living link between the training and how someone might take the relevant principles and experiences and put them into action. The group provides a safe place for experimentation, while my presence adds a little motivation. For the students this is the moment when things get real.

Sitting in the back of the room while a student delivers a talk on mindfulness or compassion, class design or proper alignment, I am always on the edge of my seat. I am willing this person to be successful with my whole being and allowing them to make the mistakes they must make to learn what they came to learn. The joy I feel as the student inevitably shines brighter than anyone could have expected is second to none. Deeply connected to another human being, I am right there with an open mind and an open heart.

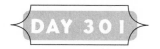

What to Bring

Humans need to practice equanimity and joy because we see things backward. If others are successful we feel like it's somehow bad for us. Maybe there's only a finite amount of success, and if someone else succeeds there will be nothing left for me.

Because of our conditioning, the path forward seems to go back and the path into light seems dark. We must learn to endure our fear with equanimity, to be able to practice compassion, loving-kindness, and joy. Each time we have a genuine opportunity to give voice to the wisdom and compassion in our hearts, a backward part of us feels afraid. These are the moments when our practice can change the course of our lives. Being right there, we can know our fear for what it is and choose to express our core values and beliefs instead. Rather than bringing a little more fear into the world, we can bring a little more love.

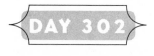

Joy as an Open Mind

Mindfulness is both spacious awareness and the awareness of being aware. It is also the spirit of adventure, the desire to learn more, the child's curiosity as she expands her discovery of the natural world in her backyard into an adult inquiry into what is true. The practice of joy reawakens our natural interest in things we do not know and have not thought or felt before. Finding joy in my daughter's success in school, science fairs, and theater has brought me into worlds that I had not known existed, and the appreciation I have for my peers working in yoga keeps me open to new ways of teaching.

As I was sitting quietly this morning, right there at the beginning of the in-breath, I felt the contracted states I have held in my body. I could feel the dread, the sadness, the craving, and the proving. I felt this history in my body as tension that I could release. Not only did it feel good to be able to let go of this tension, it put the concept of "history" in my body into perspective. Maybe history in my body is not something to be afraid of. Maybe it isn't permanent. This was a joyful experience. Then I got curious—how else was I holding history?

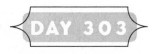

Joy as an Example

I told my friend Kevin that I was meditating with my son, Dylan, in the mornings before school. He said that must be a huge moment for a parent. I said, no, it was more about Dylan than about my ability to teach him something. Then Kevin said, "No, I mean that he was able to see what it has done for you. That what he saw meditation doing for you was good enough that at eight years old he wanted to try it." It took me a moment to fathom what Kevin's joy for my family had made clear to him. Then I smiled and said yes, it was a huge moment for me as a parent that my son would respect meditation because of my example. But what I was feeling was how price-less it is to have a friend who can feel real joy when you are successful.

PRACTICING EQUANIMITY AND JOY

1) Practice being "right there" during moments of praise and blame, gain and loss. Become the sky that holds the weather of praise and blame, gain and loss, without getting lost in it.
2) Commit to no longer making a burden of your duties.
3) Enjoy the happiness and success of others as if your own happiness depends on it.

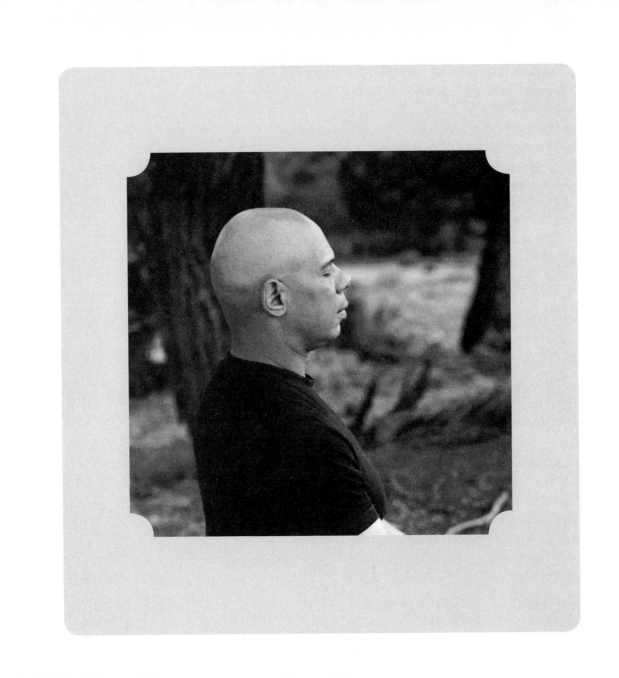

CHAPTER SEVEN

INTENTION AND BEING

The best things in life are impossible to put into words. That's the case when I try to describe why this title, and why this chapter, are so important. My life was empty of being and now it's not. My life was empty of intention and now it's not. I have known the suffering of the truly lost and now I do not. If I had not experienced it firsthand, I could not believe one life held such contrast. This is the value I bring into the world: the sure knowledge that we can be in one place and learn to live into another one.

The way we unlearn the habit of suffering is through a process of spiritual practice. I teach yoga because it is an excellent spiritual practice that is free of politics and religion. Wisdom and compassion are not religious or political; they are human. I am not against politics or religion—I am for spiritual practice. Yoga teaches two basic skills: effortless ongoing present-moment awareness (being) and effortless ongoing creation (intention). As the title of this book suggests, I believe the practices of intention and being are complementary and when practiced together manifest the full promise of yoga.

Being practices address the root cause of human suffering—our mind-made disconnect from the present moment. The traditional practices of yoga are embodied trainings in which we access the present moment through the felt experience of our bodies. Our goal-oriented way of living often misses the point of these elegantly simple practices. We cannot pour our attention into the soles of our feet and into mind-made suffering at the same time. The brain, like the body, forms around what it is repeatedly asked to do. Just as a tennis player gets better at hitting a ball the more she does it, when we repeatedly bring our attention into the body, the brain develops to support that ability. When we repeatedly offer loving-kindness, the left side of our prefrontal cortex—the part of the brain associated with empathy and happiness—measurably thickens. The practices of yoga teach us to unlearn the habits of suffering while systematically developing the habits of mindfulness and compassion.

Being practices flow from concentration, where we are learning to *be* right there, to meditation, where we are learning to *see* what's there. Mindfulness bridges the gap from one-pointed concentration to present-moment awareness. The applications for being practice are as diverse as the instances in which you are here and the number of times it is now. Grounded in the felt experience of the present moment, we awaken our true intelligence and our capacity for empathy, imagination, intuition, insight, and resilience.

When we return to the present moment, we undergo an awakening at every level of our being. We experience a physical and emotional well-being that we had not thought possible as our hearts and minds open and begin to communicate. We realize that we have been hoping that skill in *doing* can offer us what only skill in *being* can accomplish. Skill in being delivers us to an entirely new way of understanding our world, our purpose, and ourselves. Our imagination awakens and gives rise to authentic desires, desires become dreams, dreams become visions, and our vision matures into powerfully held intentions for ourselves and for our world.

I first learned about intention twenty years ago, from the writings and lectures of Deepak Chopra. At the time I was using his book *The Seven Spiritual Laws of Success* as a manual for living and attending his talks whenever he was in New England. The lessons he offered concerning what Wayne Dyer calls "the power of intention" completely changed my understanding of the flow of power in a human life. Up until that point I had thought power depended on money, organizations, governments, family, societal connections, class, special abilities, popularity, and the color of one's skin. Chopra's teachings on intention changed all of that.

What I learned from him is that a person can take her heart's desire and focus it into a specific intention. Held steadily, that intention will act upon the universe until it is fulfilled. I have experimented with this concept for two decades and during that time my life has slowly come to reflect its truth.

The implications of Chopra's teachings on intention are far reaching. To begin with, they show us that we need to put a lot of attention into the stories we have created about where the power to live the life we were born to live comes from. Intention's ability to organize its own fulfillment places on us the responsibility to make choices based not on how we believe things could happen but on what our heart's desires actually are. Living from intention is never boring and it's something that never ends.

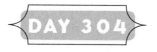

Dancing Turtles

A few days before my sister died of an overdose, I noticed that there were stickers of dancing turtles on the rear window of her car, an expression of her enthusiasm for the lifestyle practices that had grown up around the Grateful Dead. I had aspired to finding myself in this world but had only succeeded in getting high. Standing by my sister's car, I experienced a flash of insight. I came to the understanding that a practice we choose to live by is not a small thing. It's something we are going to pay a price for, whether we know it or not.

The practice I was living by at the time was quite different from the one my sister had embraced. It was just people helping other people at meetings in church basements, but it was an honest practice; you were either drinking or you were not. Some of the people at twelve-step meetings are honest and some are not, but sobriety is an honest practice. As I walked toward the passenger door of my sister's car, I could feel no honesty in the practice she was placing her faith in. The practices of being are honest. Some of the people who practice them are honest and some are not, but the experiences themselves are honest. We are either with our breath or we are not. We are either reflecting on the mind or we are reacting from it. Each time we step onto our mat or take our seat on our cushion, an honest practice is being made available to us. We have the chance to meet the moment honestly. Walking toward my sister's car, I knew it mattered that the practices of your life be honest ones.

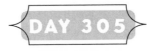

Being Awake

I think it's a mistake to sell yoga with images of skinny people in fancy poses and stories of altered states and special abilities. Even the term "enlightenment" doesn't feel right, when what the Buddha actually offered was a practical response to suffering and a means of ending it. The Buddha described himself as being "awake," which seems much more approachable to me. Becoming awake is something all of us know we can choose for ourselves. It feels like an appropriate intention as we step onto our mat or take our seat, to dedicate our practice and our life to not missing the point. Choosing to be awake is a path of courage and compassion that honors both ourselves and the blessings of this life we have been given.

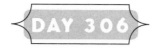

DAY 306

Being Honest

The first thing you learn within a system of oppression is to be dishonest—to say whatever you need to say and be whoever you need to be to avoid the consequences of doing otherwise. Avoiding consequences becomes the measure of an action's worth and the truth becomes irrelevant. Oppression distorts reality to the point that our lives are lived backward. The truth is denied and the lie is embraced. Throughout human history the vast majority of us have lived within oppressive systems and we have developed an ambivalent relationship to the practice of honesty.

Being honest gets a lot of positive play in our myths and our movies, but when push comes to shove—when faced with the consequences we want to avoid—we have learned to be practical. The truth becomes just a pleasant fiction, which is to say that we have learned to perpetuate oppression.

Being practices are not complicated. They do not need us to be special. They just need us to be honest, to live honestly. When we step onto our mat or take our seat we will succeed if we can be honest with ourselves. Being honest in our practice we learn the practical, transformative nature of honesty as a universal behavior. We learn how it can transform our relationship to the present moment, to the people in our lives, and to ourselves. A being practice invites us to live into the truth, to become the living possibility of liberation.

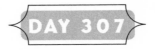

Making a Beginning

If we are being honest with ourselves, we are not here very often. We are mostly caught up in our opinions about the world, its inhabitants, and what we want from it. I do not believe it helps to pathologize the fact that our default setting is "the story of me," but I do believe we should be honest about it—and about the consequences of this self-absorption. We experience these consequences the moment we sit quietly on our meditation cushion and attempt to be right there at the beginning of the in-breath. To be right there, we have to wade through an endless stream of thoughts, and thoughts about our thoughts. Initially it feels impossible to exist outside of this stream of consciousness. And if we are honest with ourselves, we are not really trying. We've never known anything else, and we don't think we particularly want to. So we have to rely on an honest effort. We can be right there for an honest effort and an honest appraisal of what we discover. If we are honest with ourselves, we can glimpse the space between our thoughts and the space around our thoughts. If we are honest with ourselves, we do have moments of being right there; they just don't last long. If we are honest with ourselves, it is our deepest desire to be here, and every once in a while we are.

A New Pair of Shoes

An honest effort at being present on our mats and on our cushions reveals an ability to be here in a way that is entirely different from our usual approach of having one foot in the present and one foot in a cloud of thoughts (and thoughts about thoughts). We discover that there is a self we can move into that is calm and wise, heartfelt and insightful. Moving into this aspect of our being brings with it a heightening of our senses and a sharpening of our perceptive abilities. We are at once more connected to the world around us and to the world within us. At first this may last for only moments at a time—flashes of being here in a yoga class or a moment or two on our cushion—but it is a moment when we are no longer doing meditation, we are being meditation.

These glimpses of present-moment awareness are early breakthroughs. Their significance is not that they are happening (they have always been happening), it's that we are aware of them and can begin to move back into them on purpose. These flashes of present-moment awareness are like a new pair of shoes, for a new way of walking on the earth and standing in your life.

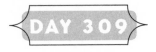

Kensho

Our first glimpses of being here are precious. They lift the burden on our hearts and provide an incentive for the diligent practice that will be asked of us. My early years of yoga were filled with moments of awareness. They had a flavor. There was the intense consciousness of the world around me: the smell of bark, the moisture in the breeze on my skin, and the timeless experience of birdsong in the distance. There was a heart-stopping sense of waking up to find myself in the home I had been seeking all my life. A sense of things being okay, and a profound desire to live a life that reflected the understanding that had been revealed.

In Japanese, these moments of clarity are called *kensho*. "*Ken*" means "seeing," and "*sho*" means "nature" or "essence." *Kensho* is when we see into the true nature—the essence—of things. The Yoga Sutras state that for those who seek, the divine is near. *Kensho* is our first proof of this, and it gives us a taste of what being here means. It gives us a reason to make an honest effort.

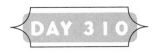

Being Afraid

Before I got sober I might have been afraid a lot, but it did not cause me to suffer that much. If I was uncomfortable, I would drink or take drugs, or move into a more comfortable contracted state, like blame, anger, or fantasy. I even came to seek out fear as a form of escape. I became an adrenaline junkie, addicted to the intensity of truly terrifying situations. While jumping out of an airplane at night or walking onto a wrestling mat, I had no other concerns. The other ways my mind created suffering were temporarily suspended while something overwhelmingly intense absorbed my attention.

Sober, I could no longer lie to myself about how things felt. Sober, I was stuck with the many ways I was afraid and the need to work honestly with this fear. There were a number of years in which I tried to talk around my fear or explain it away. This was an unrewarding process. My teachers did not get into it with me; they just asked me to bring my attention into my body and my breath. As I learned to do this I began to see the true nature of things. I saw that I was the sky and my fear was the weather. Just as the sky is not the weather, nor does it need to respond to the weather, neither was I my fear—nor did I need to be defined by it. It is enough for the sky to hold the weather effortlessly with wisdom and compassion as it passes through.

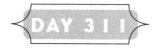

DAY 311

Being Lost

We generate delusional perceptions and contracted emotional states the way clouds generate rain. For instance, I make a comment about something, then believe that this statement is a part of me. Someone agrees with my comment—*my self*—and I am happy, full of good feelings. Someone disagrees with my comment—*my self*—and I am angry, full of negativity. Caught up in a jumble of delusional perceptions and contracted emotional states, I fight to preserve a self that does not exist. I become lost in a maze in which I cannot tell what is real and what is not.

My practice does not try to tell me which turn to take in my delusional maze. It asks me to reach down and touch the earth, to feel the grass beneath my fingers and the breeze against my cheek, the rise and fall of the breath within my chest. My practice is not there to help me escape my maze; it teaches me that there is no maze in the first place.

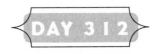

Touching the Earth

When the Buddha took his seat with the intention to awaken from his mind-made prison and bring an end to his suffering, the God of Death came to him and asked him what right he had to make such a choice. The Buddha is said to have kept his silence and simply reached down and touched the earth. He reached down and touched something real.

Each time I come back into my body, into my breath, and into the present moment I feel as though I am doing the same. There is no God of Death in my story, only the habits of my mind and my penchant for forgetting who I really am. Each time I touch the earth I remember. Standing in a yoga pose, I touch the earth. Taking a deep, slow breath on my meditation cushion, I touch the earth. Saying "I love you" to my wife, I touch the earth. Each time I touch something real I remember that we do not have the right to awaken—we are the possibility of awakening itself.

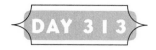

This Place

When the Buddha touched the earth he was saying, "This place. I will awaken here. I will not say that there is someplace better than where I stand. I will look to the earth beneath my feet for the path that leads to the life I choose. I will find what I need here. I have the power to choose, and when I use that power this place becomes the place where I love, where I create, where I learn, where I teach, where I find, where I let go, where I live with joy, where I die with honor, where I awaken."

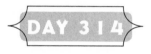

I Choose Now

When the Buddha touched the earth he was saying, "I choose now. I will not give the power of this moment away to the past or to the future. I choose now. I do not need more time, or less time, or another time. I choose now. I do not need to be more or to be less; I choose the person I am. I choose now. I do not need a golden age, an age of reason, or a romantic period. I choose now. It is enough for me to have this body, this breath, this moment. I choose now. I have the power to choose this moment, and when I use that power this moment becomes the moment I remember who I am. Each time I touch the earth this moment becomes the moment I awaken."

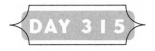

Being Wise

Being wise is like being wet when it rains. It's a part of something larger. Like the wetness of rain an entire universe has conspired to have us understand. Countless beings have given their lives to understanding so that we can understand. Countless hearts have loved well and completely, their love forming a path that leads to the earth beneath our feet. Our own suffering has been an eternity of loss and sorrow, whose darkness formed a gentle cloak to shade our hearts as they have grown and found their way to love. Our practice has been like water to the flower of our hearts. Then, one day, we look upon another person and we see ourselves. When we see their pain we see our own pain. When we see their fear we see our own fear. When we see their pride we see our own pride. When we see their love and kindness we see our own love and kindness. Like someone who was dry a moment ago and is now wet with rain, one moment we saw two, and then we saw one.

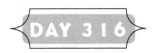

Learning to Be

The first step toward the bliss of being is recognizing that we are not experiencing it. The formation of the self that takes place during childhood is so compelling to us that the space within which it takes place and the felt sense of that space just do not matter that much. I moved my family to a remote spot on the Northern California coastline so that my children would grow up in a silence and stillness that held the sound of the ocean meeting the shore. At seven my daughter asked for a white noise machine for her bedroom because the silence freaked her out. She now sleeps without it, but you get the point—young people have other things on their minds than the bliss of being.

By the time we are adults struggling with stress and burnout we are almost incapable of understanding that the root of our problem is an inability to be here. Suffering from the disease of more, we try to cure ourselves with more—more money, more sex, more attention, more success, more productivity, more privilege, more stimulation, more food, more strife, more speed, more cults, more intensity, more dead ends. When that doesn't work we often become cynical, distrusting "alternative" medicine and the like, preferring the suffering we know to the quackery we don't. We can't solve a problem we do not know we have. This has been the key to the success of yoga in the U.S. and elsewhere. It has brought the bliss of being in the back door, disguising it in the form of an exercise class. Resting at the end of class, the student remembers what it is like to just be.

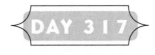

DAY 317

Placing Our Attention

Once we have rediscovered the experience of being, we begin looking for it everywhere in our lives. Is it on a golf course? Is it in a glass of wine? Is it in large sums of money, or importance, or in someone's love? Is it in a new line of work? In a life that has been about doing, it makes sense that something of value would be something new to do. This line of inquiry tends to lead to even more suffering and we start to think we might be looking in the wrong places. We keep coming back to our mats because, invariably, that is where we encounter being. One ordinary morning, our teacher guides us through some breath work—being right there as we breathe in and being right there as we breathe out. It's not anything we don't do every time we come to class, but this time, as we follow the cues, we see how they are shifting our attention and how this shifting of the attention has a power. We can see that we are always right there with something. Much of what we have been right there with no longer serves us but we did not know we had a choice. On this morning we see, for what feels like the first time, that placing our attention on something is a choice.

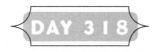

The Mind Is a Mirror

As we first learn to place our attention on the body, the breath, and the moment, our yoga practice is in a honeymoon period. We discover the pleasures of being here and it's really awesome. Sitting quietly, or resting at the end of an asana class, we feel the intensity with which we have yearned for the bliss of being. These moments of coming home are jarringly juxtaposed with the moments we spend contracting back around anger and fear, wanting and not wanting. This contrast grabs our attention. The practice of mindfulness is something we are ready to give ourselves to, and as our practice of it deepens we begin to unravel cause and effect. If we place our attention on discord, our mind will be in discord. If we place our attention on peace, our mind will be in peace. We discover that the mind is a mirror that reveals the nature of whatever we have chosen to pay attention to.

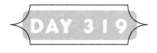

Leaves in the Wind

Sitting quietly resting in the felt experience of the body and the breath, we begin to understand the nature of our inner life. There is a calm open space that appears to be an aspect of the infinity from which we came. It has a timeless, eternal feel to it. Then there are the sounds and sensations that arise and pass within that open space. These sounds and sensations come and go within us the way things come and go in a park while we are sitting on a park bench. In fact my meditation teachers would like it if I spent my time on my cushion more like someone on a park bench than someone trying to be a "meditator." They think I would learn more and suffer less. Thoughts come and go like people walking through the park. And each thought stirs up a reaction as if it were a person walking by our bench. What sort of person is she? Do we like what she is wearing? Do we approve of how she is walking through our park?

Sitting quietly resting in the felt experience of the body and the breath, we notice that our thoughts stir our emotions like a breeze stirring leaves. When we are suffering, our emotions have been stirred this way like leaves by a breeze. This helps us to understand the meaning of *nirodha*, to be able to see without causing a stir. How could we sit like someone on a park bench watching the world go by without causing a stir?

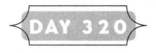

Feeling

I had spent a number of years fruitlessly trying to become present when I first heard Eckhart Tolle speak. Instead of telling us to become present, he told the audience to feel into the present moment. I am sure my teachers had been telling me to do this for years, but it wasn't until Tolle said it out loud that it made sense to me. Feeling into the present was something I already knew how to do. I knew how to taste soup and feel the temperature of the water in a pool without thinking about it. I knew how to shift my attention from thinking to feeling.

Once I began to explore the present moment in this way, I realized I had found a way to be present without internal commentary. I was able to feel without judging, to be right there for the felt experience of a breath or the near-silent beat of my heart. These moments did not last very long but I understood what they meant. I had the ability to be present for the world around me without getting lost in it, without causing a stir.

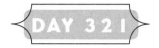

Knowing

Being available to life without commentary frees us from the possibility of mind-made suffering. There is no mental wind to stir the emotions. The relief this brings to us after decades of reacting to our reactions is worth whatever trouble it might take. It's a beautiful form of peace that we are bringing into our life and from which we develop the ability to see, feel, taste, smell, and hear without commentary. It would be enough.

Sitting quietly resting in the felt experience of the body and the breath, we become available for the experience of life without the effort of commentary. In the absence of commentary, new things enter into our awareness that have previously been outside our perception. In the absence of commentary, our true capacity to know what our senses—and what our physical, emotional, and energetic bodies—are telling us is revealed. We start to actually see the person in front of us and to hear what they are saying and what they are not saying. In the clear open space of the peace we find in the present moment, we rediscover our capacity to know what is true.

CHAPTER SEVEN

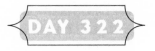

Knowing More and Doing Less

The world of doing is busy and loud and the people who live there like it that way. In the world of doing, noise and agitation mean things are getting done. In the world of knowing, things tend to get done with silence and stillness. Patience turns out to be a real go-getter with a capacity for getting things done that almost nothing else matches. In the world of knowing, we are happy to live without many of the things that are needed in the world of doing. In fact, very few things turn out to be absolutely necessary, which saves us a lot of time and energy. In the world of knowing, listening is necessary, as are learning to forgive, saying "I love you," laughing, and spending time on activities whose only purpose is the experience of joy. The world of doing cares only for what can be seen; the world of knowing flows from the unseen world of being. The people who live in the world of knowing love what can be seen because they know where it comes from and where it is going. In the world of knowing, nobody ever does anything—yet everything gets done.

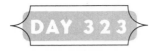

The Sunset Room

The main building of the Kripalu Center for Yoga & Health has four floors. At the center of the fourth floor is a room called the Sunset Room because of the view it provides of the sun setting over the ridges and valleys of Western Massachusetts. One summer, I spent six weeks watching the sun set from this room. The years before had been marked by trauma and addiction, sobriety and recovery, love and loss. I was learning to be a yoga teacher and preparing for a life that would become progressively empty of the suffering I had always known, and full of challenges I could not then imagine. Sitting quietly watching the sun set, I did not know any of this. I knew how it felt to be still as the world transformed around me. I knew the way darkness fell without a sound. I knew how the air changed as it cooled. I knew what it felt like to be here and nowhere else. I knew that it mattered that I had found this sunset, these colors, and this air. I knew that I was creating my future by learning to love being here.

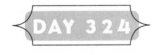

Being Attached

When we are attached to something we feel like we have a purpose, a reason to get out of bed in the morning. Attachments give us a future and a past, something to look forward to and something to look back on. Attachments lend shape and scale to our lives; they give us direction, so that we know where we are going and we know we are going to get there soon. Clinging to our preferences has given humanity a world to live in, a world that revolves around us, a world we feel we can almost control. This world never changes, and if we don't leave it behind, neither do we—we're forever grasping after a vanishing world where we never have to stop being afraid.

Some of us leave this world for good in one big whoosh, but most of us go back and forth between the experience of being and the experience of attachment. It's a tricky period because attachment makes sense to us when we are attached. We can get caught up in it for years at a time. This is why we need a practice—something that we can keep coming back to— to remind us that we can stop being afraid and stop making a world small enough for our fear.

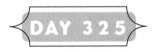

DAY 325

Being Great

I have the habit of attachment and I am often unable to see how attachment is shrinking my world. Over the years, I have embraced the practice of finding joy in others' achievements to help me when my world has gotten small. Seeing others live without fear helps me move beyond my own.

There is a story in my family about my father-in-law's friend Bert Moore, who brought Martin Luther King Jr. to Southern Methodist University to speak in 1966. While an undergrad, Bert fought and won an uphill battle to bring the civil rights leader to a city that was still segregated. There's a picture of Bert sitting behind MLK as he speaks to three thousand students. It's a simple image of greatness. Fifty years later, the story and the image inspire the purest form of joy in me. Joy for Bert's courage and vision. Joy for Martin Luther King's greatness. Joy for the ability of one person's greatness to inspire greatness in others. When I hold a joy this big, I find it difficult to fit back into the world of my attachments.

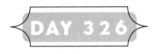

The Greatness of Being

The simplest way out of the small, cramped world of my attachments is to move into the spacious experience of being. Yoga makes this pretty accessible. It teaches us to know the body in the body, to know the breath in the breath, and to know the moment in the moment. It makes the bliss of being something we can move into effortlessly.

There is a danger that we might make yoga into a new identity or religion, but if we keep it simple and just keep coming back to this body, this breath, this moment, we'll find an alternative to the world of our attachments. We'll find the depths of our own hearts and as many ways to say "I love you" as there are stars in the sky. We'll find the true nature of our mind and as many ways to understand our world as there are breaths in a lifetime. We'll find the true nature of this body, this breath, this living planet, and as many paths to travel as there are trees in a forest. We'll know this moment and find all the time we need.

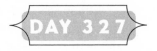

The Path of Least Resistance

The unmanifest holds what physicists call the "matrix of possibility," which is to say, all that is possible and all that is impossible. Like water flowing downhill, the unmanifest seeks the path of least resistance. If we present it with our karmic patterns it will pour itself into them, continually manifesting family dramas and traumas one generation after the next. If we present the unmanifest with our hearts' desires, it will pour itself into them, continually manifesting our dreams and visions year after year. Mindfulness and compassion allow us to deconstruct the negative blueprints the unmanifest has been expressing through us. Intention allows us to construct positive ones.

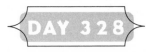

Eighty-eight Keys

Our consciousness forms the link between the limited and the unlimited, and through conscious intent we have the ability to guide the process of creation.

The piano has a finite number of keys, yet musicians can compose an infinite number of songs on them. The English alphabet has a finite number of letters, yet poets can write an infinite number of poems with them.

Numbers on a chalkboard exist in two dimensions, yet scientists have been able to use them to plot a course across the stars and through the solar system. The limitations of our world offer the limitless the possibility of form. Our imaginations offer the limitless an endless number of worlds to create.

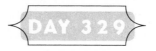

Cambridge Young People's Meeting

The year I got sober my sister died. It took me several years to process and integrate this combination of experiences. My first years sober were spent in simple jobs where I could leave work at work. I rode my bike, went to twelve-step meetings, had dinner with friends, ran a marathon in DC and a couple more in New York. It was a good time in my life. After five years sober, I took my first job that would need me to be mentally and emotionally present. It was a stretch. I was a counselor for children with emotional disorders and I was their substance abuse specialist, which meant I ran their substance abuse group and took them to twelve-step meetings.

Taking teenagers to twelve-step meetings is more than a little stressful. My kids were constantly trying to sneak off to get high or have sex. One of their excuses for doing what they would have done anyway was that the people at the meetings were "old," meaning over eighteen. This was true, so I started a twelve-step meeting in Cambridge down the street from our treatment center for young people. It was the first time I tried to put what Deepak Chopra teaches about intention into action. I would have to be the link between the manifest world and the unmanifest world. Beyond the practicalities of setting up these meetings, what I really did was hold an intention steadily and see if it arranged its own fulfillment. It did. Seventeen years later you can still find young people getting sober at eight P.M. on Wednesday night in Central Square in Cambridge, Massachusetts.

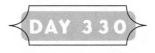

A Basement in Michigan

I wrote my first book so that people who were beginning to choose spiritual solutions for their problems would have a little company and a little guidance during those early years. I saw the secret vulnerability of this time in life. The beginning of such a path is precious and precarious and the window of opportunity is often brief. I wrote *Meditations from the Mat* to be a support in an hour of need. That was the intention I held.

Seven years later I was leading a teacher training in the Santa Cruz Mountains and a young woman from Michigan came to me with a story. She had given my book to her sister but had not yet found yoga herself. At the end stage of her addiction she was helping her sister move and found my book in a basement on a quiet afternoon. She stopped packing and sat down to read it. Two years later, she was clean and sober and attending my teacher training. She told me my book was a support to her as she worked to make a new life for herself. She may not have known it, but she was also reminding me that the intentions we hold are transmitted through the actions we take.

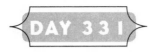

DAY 331

The California Coastline

In 2002, I began writing about a house that I wanted to live in on the California coast. It was beautiful and warm all year round and roomy enough to provide guests with a place to stay. I did not know anything about the California coast. But that's what I wanted. I'd had enough of cities and I wanted to be somewhere rural, by the sea.

I knew that I wanted it to be in a college town with a lot of cool movie theaters and restaurants. I wanted palm trees and white-sand beaches. I wanted quiet forests where I could take endless walks with my dog. I wanted good public schools and a strong sense of community. I agonized that all of this might not be impossible. It seemed like a huge change from the life I was already living, which was formed around a business, a house, and a family.

I kept writing about my dream house. The years went by, and my intention for myself and my family held. On New Year's Day 2007, I wrote in my diary that I wanted to move my family to my ideal location by May 2008. That fall, in an effort to make something happen, my wife went to Oakland to look at spaces for a yoga studio. Oakland didn't quite fit my vision, but I could see how I could make a studio there work. But my wife never got to Oakland. For the one and only time in her life, her back went out and she had to stay in bed when she got to California. Each day I called her to see how things were going. Each day she said she was still at her dad's place in Santa Cruz, a beachy college town that borders a vast redwood forest on California's rural central coastline. On the third day we talked on the phone for a while and she told me about the bodyworkers who were helping her, then I asked her, "How's Santa Cruz?" The following spring we celebrated my son Dylan's second birthday at his grandmother's house in Boston and left the next day for our new life in California. We arrived on May 20, 2008.

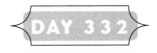

Writing It Down

In the fall of 1994, I read a chapter in a book by Deepak Chopra that said I should write down my heart's desires and keep them on my person, taking them out once in a while to reflect on their felt experience. I was praying daily and getting miraculous results, so the idea that a scrap of paper in my wallet could somehow influence the course of events did not seem as far-fetched as it sounds.

I wrote my list and kept it in my wallet. I reflected on it once in a while but within six months I no longer needed to, because I was living it already.

DAY 333

Being Teachable

I grew up without any conscious connection to the unmanifest—no religion, no sense of spirit, just a love of dogs and a love of sports. The closest thing I had to a spiritual experience was the sense that my life was out of control. I was an addict doomed to an addict life, and that, apparently, was that. My powerlessness was so loud that until I got sober it was all there was; it was my only relationship. Just me and what was killing me.

When I got sober I realized that I did not know anything about anything. I had just spent the last twelve years locked in a closet with my addiction. I joined a community that helped me figure out what had happened to me and what to do next. This had the effect of making learning my full-time job. I had to learn everything, from how to pay a bill to how to nod your head when someone is speaking to you so that they know you are listening. It also meant that learning was a matter of life and death. If I could not learn I was going back into the closet and I was probably not coming out this time. I became teachable with my whole heart and soul. I learned what would get me dead first: thinking I knew when I did not. I saw all kinds of people die that way. You can't learn something you think you already know. I developed the ability to become empty of thinking that I knew. Learning was survival; intellectual pride was not. Life happens in this moment, and this moment has never happened before. Being teachable is the practice of meeting life, this unprecedented moment, knowing that you do not know.

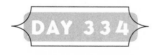

Not Knowing as Freedom and Joy

Once the initial shock of getting sober died down a little and I settled into a perpetual state of astonishment and gratitude, I began to see how my world

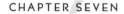

had changed. Not knowing meant that anything was possible. In fact, any-thing was *probable*. The years ahead of me had to be filled with something—why not wonder, adventure, courage, and love?

My imagination was quietly pardoned, cleared of all charges, and set free. Not knowing opened the door to wisdom and let my teachers in. In the open space of not knowing, my mind has grown sharper and more spacious each year and my heart has never tired of a life where I never know what I can do until I try.

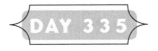

Verified Faith

My teachers use the term "verified faith" to refer to the direct experience of a principle we have placed our faith in and practiced properly effecting the positive change that we were told it would. We cannot verify our faith in a principle until we have applied it. My faith in not knowing has had countless moments of verification. Some of these moments have a practi-cal quality to them—moments when I do not stick my foot in my mouth even though every cell in my body mistakenly thinks it "knows," or when knowing that I do not know allows me to take practical and necessary risks with people or in business. Some moments have made my spiritual maturity possible when nothing else could, such as when I chose to take one more step toward forgiveness even though I "knew" it was hopeless.

Then there are the truly critical moments when not knowing opens doors that must be opened for me to live the life I am here to live. The moment I said yes to the opportunity to teach yoga was like that. The moment I said yes to my first meditation retreat was like that. The moment I was willing to see the connection between getting clear about my heart's desires and the course my life has taken was like that too.

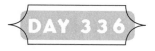

Honest, Open-minded, and Willing

A key part of the twelve-step program is HOW, a way to approach your life based on the spiritual principles of honesty, open-mindedness, and willingness. These virtues are recited at the beginning of many meetings, and as the years passed, they seeped into my worldview. I learned to trust these virtues and be wary when I moved away from them. Meeting life honestly, with an open mind and a willing heart, felt like a humble form of courage, the kind of courage I was learning that life requires.

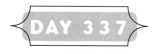

Direction

When I first read Deepak Chopra, I simply followed his instructions and based whether I was going to continue to follow them on the results they yielded. The results were good, so good that I have followed his instructions on intention ever since. I did not make an identity out of these instructions or the results. I did not make a religion out of them, either. I was simply honest with myself and willing to choose the best.

What I found in those pages could fill any number of books. I learned that I never know what's really on my mind and in my heart until I write it down. That there are hopes and dreams hovering right below the surface of my awareness that rise up to be seen when I put pen to paper. Once something is on paper, I look at it from every angle and make a conscious decision to choose what I have written. Having a list of my desires feels like setting a course, pointing my life in a direction. I can choose the direction I want my life to go in, sit down, check in with myself, and point my life in the direction of my heart's desires. I have learned that writing down my intentions has the same effect as choosing a route for a cross-country drive. Before long the names on the map become places you have been.

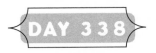

Leadership

It was not long after I started writing down my heart's desires that I first began having significant influence in other people's lives. There might be low-stakes leadership positions, but I have never had one. Whenever people count on me, it matters to them how I handle my responsibilities. Being responsible is being accountable, and being accountable creates a healthy sort of pressure in our life. I began learning how to be a leader in the military and had a chance to watch a lot of people under pressure. Pressure tends to give us tunnel vision, which in turn causes us to make choices without a complete grasp of the situation. Leaders need to maintain excellent situational awareness and having a plan is a good start. The military taught me to write down a very clear order of operations for the people I led, and social work taught me to write down a very clear treatment plan for my clients, so it was no surprise that writing down my heart's desires was similarly helpful. Having a plan organizes what you are trying to accomplish. True situational awareness includes a plan, certainly, but also includes the why.

The military had a special word for the why of a mission: it was the mission's *intent*. As a military officer I was trained not only to understand the specifics of my mission but also to be clear on the overall intent of the mission. How did the mission fit into my commander's overall vision? Holding the larger vision in mind while attending to and communicating effectively about the in-the-moment details is a true test of leadership. For the last twenty years, I have been in one leadership situation after the next, and writing down my broader goals—my intent—has made it possible to stay rooted in the why of what I am doing even as I attend to the how.

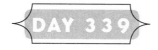

Imagination as Leadership

Successful day-to-day leadership is all about effective communication. Are the people we lead clear about the who, what, when, and where of what is required of them? Different people hear things differently, they learn things differently, so we can never be sure if our message has been heard. To make matters more complicated people learn at different rates at different times.

Studies have shown that when people are under stress, they do significantly less well on standardized testing than when they are not under stress. Reality testing—checking back with people about what they think is expected of them—is highly recommended, and I find that having people do the same thing a bunch of times works best. Sooner or later everyone gets on the same page. There is an element of brute force, a willingness to instill knowledge through sheer repetition, about getting groups to understand something. This sort of work tends to make leaders rigid, stuck to systems that have proven to be effective in the past, regardless of whether they are relevant in the present. Caught up in rationalizing the relevance of an approach we are comfortable with, we lose touch with our creative impulse.

Situational awareness includes our imagination. As much as leaders are counted on to get things done, they are also counted on to hold the larger vision. To stay rooted in their imagination, to stay inspired and open to new ways of being successful. Writing down my heart's desires and reflecting on them often has made it possible for me to maintain my intention to be a visionary leader as well as a productive one.

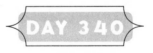

Believing

I tell yoga students that our own experience is the manual we are given to understand what it is to be a human being. I tell them that we are meant to learn about one another by learning about ourselves, and that as we come to know our own sorrows and infatuations, our own strengths and confusions, we are gaining insight into the lives of those around us. My manual has revealed that anyone, with the right support, can achieve pretty much anything. I went into my work with others knowing this about people because I knew it about myself.

To effectively lead people you must genuinely believe they can do what you are asking them to do. It also helps if you believe in people in general, if your understanding of them is that they will rise to any occasion, and that if they haven't yet, they will. Writing down my heart's desires and reflecting on them often has also made me a believer in the future we are all living into. When I am in a position of responsibility, I am so with an unwavering faith in the people I am leading and the future we are working toward together—a faith that has already been verified.

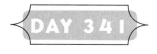

The Light Finds Us

Writing down my heart's desires and reflecting on them often helps me point my life in a direction that is aligned with my core values and beliefs. Within the space of that alignment I can let my imagination flow. I can imagine, I can dream, and I can believe. As my inner vision is drawn to a specific expression of what I want, my heart will let me know the extent to which it serves the highest good for all. A friend of mine calls the moment when your heart leaps at the prospect of a dream or vision "the surge." Another good sign is when your dreams for the future are so beautiful they make you cry—this is how I felt whenever I thought about my ideal house on the California coast. Making the time to dream and checking in with your heart about which dream gets to go to the front of the line is good living. It would be enough.

Our intentions organize their own fulfillment. Everything in this universe is information vibrating at different frequencies, and like attracts like. The information contained in our intentions forms a vibration that attracts matching vibrations. This is why we often live into the essence of our intentions rather than the actual shape and color of them. Who we are, what we believe, and how we are being will always be reflected back to us, will always be drawn to us. Mother Teresa set up shop in one of the darkest places on earth and the light found her there.

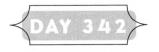

Standing in the Possibility

I worked on an ambulance for a while with a friend named Tom. He introduced me to the idea of "standing in," which referred to holding such a strong intention around something that you feel like you are standing in it. It made sense to me that a person could stand in the intention of the life they wanted and that life would grow up around them. Tom and I were both newly sober and did not have much, but you could already see the life that was beginning to grow up around us.

After work on the ambulance I often practiced yoga asana to let go of my day, and mountain pose began to feel like standing in the possibility of the life that I was choosing for myself. I could feel how much it mattered to allow myself to know and to feel exactly how I wished to stand in the world. I felt a powerful connection to myself and to others. I could feel how standing in my possibility helped everyone else stand in theirs.

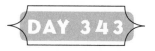

This One Thing

Eventually, I found my way to a yoga classroom and I've stayed there ever since. The years passed and I kept watching people come to class and do their best—at the end of a long day, in the midst of one, or at the beginning of one, taking some time to care for themselves, to prepare, to let go. No matter who came to my classroom, no matter what their life had contained, the way they did their poses was the way they did their life. I saw that if I could help them with how they did their yoga poses I could help them with everything. My job is helping people with this one thing: learning to stand in the possibility of the life they choose, efforting less, and feeling more. Learning to be in a yoga pose in a way that they can try again later that day on a park bench and maybe still later for a breath or two before saying "I love you" to their loved ones.

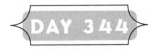

DAY 344

Holding the Pose

*Out beyond ideas of wrongdoing and right doing there is a field.
I'll meet you there.*

Rumi

The felt experience of a yoga pose is the perfect place to become acquainted with a world beyond right doing and wrongdoing. In class, I start with what we are good at. I tell the students to be strong, to feel how strong they are. And they do. Then I tell them to balance that strength with ease. Softening a little and brightening a lot, they discover the field beyond strength and ease. The same class might involve the field beyond stability and freedom, or the field beyond yes and no. Later that day a student might be able to experience the field beyond wanting and not wanting, or the field beyond good people and bad people. She knows that the field is there because she has found it for herself in class. She felt into it and knew it to be true. Swinging between right and wrong, good and bad, wanting and not wanting, feels less skillful, less desirable then the nuanced truth of the pose she felt that day. Later, as she reflects on her heart's desires and she feels the pull of hope and fear, she comes into her body and her breath and finds a place to stand, a field beyond hope and fear.

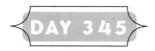

The Ideal Scene

Marc Allen has written a couple of books that have helped me refine the process of writing down my heart's desires. In one of them he asks the reader to write out her vision of a perfect life. I have embraced this concept and taught it to many people I have coached over the years. I tell my students to imagine themselves three to five years in the future and then write a short paper about the ideal life they want to be living. I tell them to open their hearts entirely, and to be willing to write down their dreams, however impossible they may feel. I encourage them to enjoy using their imagination and tell them that the details matter. How do you want things to smell? What colors do you want in your home? What does your ideal morning look like? Your ideal evening? Just stretching your imagination in this fashion, and the self-awareness that comes out of the exercise, would be enough.

Once you have your "ideal scene" written on paper, your life has changed. The Buddha said that once you know something to be true you must live up to it. You now know more about yourself than you knew before. Your attention has been drawn to colors, scents, breezes, emotions, adventures, and loves that express your heart's desire, and where your attention goes, energy flows. You now have a direction and your life will start to organize itself around it.

CHAPTER SEVEN

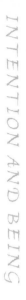

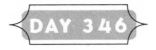

DAY 346

Life Lessons

We are going to meet the lessons life has in store for us on any road we take. The question is, what road do we want to be on when our lessons come calling? I pondered this for at least a decade before I decided I wanted life's lessons to meet me somewhere warm and green, enjoying a family life filled with happiness, joy, and laughter. I decided I wanted to meet life's lessons with the wisdom, compassion, and steadiness my teachers display every time I interact with them. I prayed that I would meet life's lessons helping others have the life I wanted for myself. I prayed that I would meet life's lessons in a way that expressed my love and gratitude for this life I have been given.

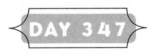

DAY 347

Yoga Is a Desire of the Heart

Writing down your heart's desires and reflecting on them often may sound good when you are stuck in a cubicle dreaming of working with kids in the mountains of Wyoming. But it sounds like just another thing you won't get around to once you're Counselor Susan in the middle of the Wyoming wilderness keeping track of addicted teens as they learn a new way of life. In the beautiful chaos of "living the dream" we can rely on the *yamas* and the *niyamas* as a simple and effective way to bring our heart's desires into our daily life. The principles of yoga articulate the place where our diverse dreams connect. Regardless of the dream, we want to act within it from a place of wisdom and compassion, courage and joy, vision and steadiness. Yoga is something to hold on to when everything else is moving.

Living into my ideal scene, I have often found myself asked to make a choice without the time, or rest, or support, or nourishment, or guidance, or resources, or options I would have preferred. I might be living my ideal scene but I am often not living my ideal circumstances when I have to make the sorts of choices that determine the future I will be living into. In those times I simply have to consider the choice before me and make the choice that expresses the principles of yoga to act in alignment with my true heart's desires. Yoga is always my true heart's desire.

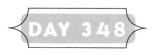

Practice Is a Desire of the Heart

Dreams are rough-and-ready things and they matter a tremendous amount to us. The stakes are high and the mistakes we make are for the best, but they will hurt a lot before we understand this. People living into their dreams attract a lot of positive attention and other people rely on them. The choices we make affect a larger and larger number of people. Constantly breaking new ground, we will have to be willing to fail over and over again in order to succeed. A life of fulfillment demands all we have and a little more. We will need a strong practice.

A practice that teaches us to be calm and still until we understand

A practice that teaches us to be kind and gentle as a matter of course

A practice that teaches us happiness, joy, and laughter

A practice that teaches us to have boundaries of steel and a heart of compassion

A practice that teaches us to stand for something while allowing others to do the same

A practice that offers the sure knowledge that we are never less alone than when we act alone for love

A practice that is our heart's desire

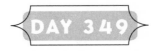

Jack

I have studied at a pair of retreat centers that were founded by meditation teachers of my parents' generation. These centers have been open for decades, providing impeccable instruction in mindfulness and compassion to tens of thousands of people every year. One of the founders is Jack Kornfield, a teacher I first encountered through his writings and have since been able to study with on a number of retreats. He is my ideal in terms of a life of practice, vision, and service. He is also the best storyteller I have ever met, which is a talent I am very fond of. When people can talk on retreat, he is affectionately and reverently referred to as Jack.

Jack has pursued his own practice with the utmost steadfastness and he has brought that practice into the ordinary trials of career and family. While attending to these priorities he has cofounded meditation centers whose aim is to share with others what has brought him so much happiness. One unique aspect of these centers is that half of each student's costs are covered by donations that Jack and his colleagues tirelessly raise year after year. Another is that Jack and his colleagues are paid by donation only. The leadership of these centers is nonhierarchical: no one person sits at the top, and the everyday teaching is always done by teams. The organization Jack has dedicated his life to supporting is truly sustainable because it is not about Jack, or anyone else; it is about the practice and the promise it holds for humanity. Jack has held a vision for himself and his world across the entire span of his adult life, a vision of wisdom and compassion, a vision of generosity and service, a vision that has effectively touched the lives of countless people, not the least of which are my wife, my children, and me. He is my ideal of a strong practice giving rise to a strong intention, and to what happens next.

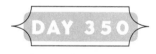

Dylan

My daughter, Jasmine, loves school. She loves the friends and the sense of community. She loves the teachers, the order, the ritual, and the challenge. She loves to learn, she loves to help others learn, she loves to succeed and loves the respect she sees in her parents' eyes when she does. She is the first child.

My son, Dylan, does as well in school as Jasmine but couldn't care less. He prefers trees and furry creatures, stories and the world of the imagination. When the players take a knee in soccer because someone is hurt, he runs to the boy or girl who is down before taking a knee so that the player is not alone.

He is a child of the heart. This fall, when school started back up, he told me he was scared and I told him he should meditate with me. He did. It's been a few weeks and so far he has found it fairly effortless and effective. He is even starting to like school a little.

After meditation last week, as I was reviewing the technique, Dylan asked, "So is relaxing the body what you are trying to do?" I said, "Yes it is, and becoming alert as well. Dylan, just remember to look for the sun and the moon. Being still and relaxed is the moon, being awake and curious is the sun. When you are wrestling, you stay calm so that you don't get tired and you can see the opportunities in a situation—that is the moon. When you are wrestling, you are fierce and determined—that is the sun. The sun and the moon together are wrestling. Look for the sun and moon in whatever you do. They will always be there."

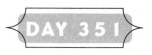

The Moon

You would think addiction is the experience of craving. It's not; it's just an in-depth education in fear and powerlessness, the primary colors of human suffering. Fear shrinks our universe. When we are afraid we contract into ourselves, losing our connection with the world around us and our ability to understand it. Fear makes any accurate sense of self impossible. To be disconnected from the truth of who we are is to feel truly powerless. When we feel powerless our values, our beliefs, our hopes, and our dreams do not matter as much as our fear and our desire to escape that feeling. The addict will trade away everything in his life for a moment of relief. The final lesson of addiction is to make you live that way day after day for years on end.

If you survive your addiction, the moon will still be there. The clouds will part and there she will be. The light of the moon is still, empty, and private. A place for wounded hearts and withered spirits to take their first steps back into a world they felt they had lost. A place to remember cool summer breezes and the ease of a good night's sleep. The moon's light is perfect for long walks under the stars. By her light we will look into eyes that love us back. Sitting with her, we will remember that there is no time, only now. With her light on our face we will leave the house of our sorrow and begin the journey of our joy.

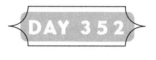

DAY 352

The Sun

You would think surrender is the experience of giving up. It's not. It's just an in-depth education in courage and honesty, the primary colors of human virtue. Courage holds life's door open for our hearts. When we live with courage our hearts are offered to the world and the world can touch them. Within the space courage provides we can live honestly. Our personal power flows from this ability; living honestly is living powerfully. When we are grounded in this form of power our values, our beliefs, our hopes, and our dreams matter more to us than our fear and our desire to escape it. The final lesson of surrender is that we must keep learning to live this way, day after day, for years on end.

If we choose to surrender, the sun will still be there. The clouds will part and there she will be. The light of the sun is warm, gentle, and strong. A place for wounded hearts and withered spirits to find the strength they need to walk back into life. A place to remember picnics by a river and the way your heart leaps at the sight of flowers in bloom. The sun's light is perfect for adventures with friends. In her presence we will take someone's hand and they will take ours. In her warmth we will remember that we can begin now always. With her light on our face we will find our place among the grateful and our love will be true.

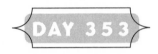

Feeling the Moon on Our Face

The mental agitation and physical stress of ordinary human suffering create so much spiritual pollution that we can no longer see the sun or the moon or take comfort in their light. Our first steps out of suffering must, therefore, be taken in the dark. We simply come to the belief that the pain of change is preferable to the pain of staying the same. As we embrace yoga as a way of making our lives a little better, we are rewarded with less drama and more order. The first buds of our own personal spring start to appear. And then, one day, we are taught to move back into the body. To be right there with the in-breath and to be right there with the out-breath. It is often after a few moments spent like this in a yoga class that we first find that we can be right there as our body starts to rest. Our breathing slows and the tension we have been holding in our bodies starts to fade. Resting in the felt experience of the body, we feel the clouds part and the moon come out. Later that

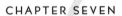

day, in the midst of the world's busyness, we step into a moment of stillness, like someone stepping into a sudden cloudburst; smiling at the wonder of it, we discover that we can find no reason to be afraid.

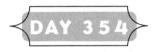

Feeling the Sun on Our Face

When we are new to yoga we need to rest for a while, like a newborn puppy. Stepping out of the world we have known all our lives and into this new one is a bit of a shock. Everything hits us a little harder. Our joy is greater, our anger burns brighter, and the grief we have been avoiding finds us unprepared. It is a time for long walks in the moonlight, to feel back into the beauty of the world around us, to be in this body, this breath, this moment. In class one day the teacher offers a new pose, one that makes us afraid, but we try it anyway. For a moment, you are upside down, balancing with the strength of your arms, balancing with the strength of your concentrated mind, the strength of your courage and determination. Coming out of the pose, you can't help smiling, and you feel as if the world is smiling with you. Later that day, you feel the sun on your face and the strength of your stride. With each step you feel that life has just begun.

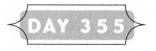

Practicing the Moon

Most years I spend ten days in silence. I practice silence in a place of great natural beauty where it's warm during the day and cool at night. The routine is pretty much the same, year after year, so I don't have to keep track of much, just sitting and walking meditation as the sun rises, stays high for while, then sets, and the moon comes out. At the end of each day, I sit on a bench and look at the moon above a couple of nearby hills. No matter how hot the day is, it usually cools at night, and there is that special smell as the landscape lets go of the day. When I first started going into silence I was in the midst of a very complicated life and my time on the bench felt like a reprieve. These days I am just happy to have the time to appreciate something so utterly beautiful. When I sit on my bench and look at the moon I no longer have a life—I am life.

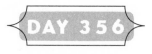

Practicing the Sun

My earliest teachers taught me to think of my work life as an aspect of my spiritual life. Initially, they said, it should provide a healthy structure for my days and a few opportunities to grow. Over time, it might begin to express my desire to serve others, but it was not necessary for that to be the case.

Work was not something to make an identity out of, and if I wished to serve others there would never be an end to the volunteer opportunities available to me. I eventually chose yoga teaching as my path of service because it felt like the best way to ensure my own continued spiritual growth. That has not always been the case, but taken as a whole I have no complaints and a lot of gratitude on this score. Yoga teaching has kept my head in the game.

When I found it, the practice of yoga was perfect in my eyes, and as a new teacher, I merely aspired to offering others what my teachers had offered me. I had a knack for it and was soon singing my song as a yoga teacher. For a while this was enough, to sing my song and to have others benefit from it. There was a loneliness to singing my song, though, that I could not shake. I thought that maybe the loneliness was part of my service—something that made teaching yoga teaching yoga—and I made an identity out of it. This did not help, and as my practice deepened, I saw the problem and understood the solution. Having a song was the problem, being a part of one was the solution. Today I do not have a song; today I am a grateful part of one, and it is perfect in my eyes.

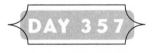

Practicing the Sun and Moon Together

Every breath we take without adding suffering lets a little more light into our lives. The light is always there; we simply need to allow it in. When we do, our minds clear, sharpen, and then become spacious and brilliant. Our bodies display astonishing resilience, regaining their former health and surpassing it now that they are partnered with a mind that is learning to let go.

Our emotional life takes a little longer to straighten out, but it has a more complex job to perform and we will be the wiser for it. Our hearts heal last but will prove to be the strongest and wisest of them all. When the heart says yes, the sun is truly shining on our faces. This is the experience of strength and purpose, vision, courage, and daring greatly. This is the experience of placing who we are at the service of life itself. This is the experience of knowing why we are here.

A love and respect for the life we have been given forms around the yes in our heart. A love and respect that expresses itself in the desire to care for the body that carries us and the heart that guides us. A desire to know peace and to feel the earth beneath our feet. After a day spent with the sun on our face, we learn to welcome the light of the moon.

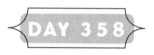

Living the Sun and Moon Together

In my thirties I knew mostly the sun. I was successful and felt like I was making up for lost time. I taught yoga most days, and my practice was a way to digest the lessons from the day before and prepare for the day ahead. Which is to say, my yoga was sun and sun. I went on vacations with my wife, whose company makes me extremely happy, but after so many years without the sun I was caught in an understandable attachment to it. Then my children were born and I began to look ahead to years of providing for them. All of a sudden, the sun felt pretty hot and the land felt pretty dry. My forties were spent learning to live with both the sun and moon together.

I was taught to plan my day around my practice, and for the last twenty-five years, I have. Each week I have a plan that attempts to create a synergistic balance of experiences. The key word in this plan is "and." It's the "and" that brings it all together. Each day features a sun practice and a moon one. I create balanced weeks by blending the moon practices of meditation and yoga with the sun practices of hiking, surfing, and a workout my friend Greg Amundson has designed for me. The sun practices fill me with the heart for the struggle and the spirit of adventure. The moon practices release the tensions held in my mind and body, reconnect me with my heart and my wisdom, and root me back into this perfect time and this beautiful place.

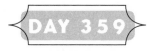

Moments

In my thirties I taught yoga. In my forties I taught yoga teachers. I also travel thirty weekends a year—year in and year out. I am a gold or silver member on a number of airlines and at a number of hotels. Looking at my life this way is overwhelming. But it is not how I live. I don't do weeks, I don't even do days; I do moments.

I have a chatty trip to the airport. Then I have a restful time as I wait to board. When I arrive at my destination, I make time to practice and to read a good book. Showering and shaving before I teach, I listen to music that reminds me how perfect yoga is in my eyes and how much I am touched by the people who show up to my classes. At the studio, I set up my harmonium and take a moment to ground the class and guide us into our breathing. Then we take our first om together and I am in the presence of my teachers. My life must be lived one moment at a time. I stay rooted in

CHAPTER SEVEN

the larger vision by writing down my heart's desires and reflecting on them often. I stay rooted in this time and this place by keeping the light of the moon on my face and the earth beneath my feet. I choose to believe that a good day is just a series of good moments, and that a good day is the best way to express my gratitude for being here.

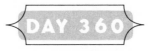

Passing on the Peace of the Moonlight

When I was twenty-eight and still in the army reserves, I went for my annual physical. My blood pressure was 140 over 90 and the doctor asked me if I came from a line of people who had died young. I was clean and sober and running marathons at the time of the checkup. It was not what I was doing that was the problem; it was how I was being. You did not have to tell me this. My childhood had been relentlessly traumatic and I had never learned how to calm down without twelve beers and half a pint of something strong. I did not know how to respond to my doctor. I did not like being in a permanent state of fight-or-flight any more than I liked living in a world where that was the only way to be.

Many people die this way, never knowing a moment free from the corrosive experience of fear. I try never to forget this. The people at twelve-step meetings taught me how to put down the drink, but it was my yoga teachers who taught me a new way to be. They taught me that it wasn't enough to change what I was doing; I needed to change how I was being as well. I began doing yoga and soon my practice was changing the way I was being— and my blood pressure. After my first yoga class I could not imagine a day without its soothing presence. After my first meditation retreat I could not imagine a life without the sanity and humanity the practice of meditation makes possible. I turned fifty this year and my blood pressure is 120 over 70, as it has been for the last twenty years. With the help of my teachers I have learned to touch the earth with my fingers as I sit in silent moonlight. It is all I need. The peace of the moonlight is enough for me. All that remains to be done is to pass it on. Pass it on with all I have, for as long as I have.

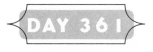

The Path of Sun and Moon

It's quite something to get a second chance at life. It's also a lot to sort out. There are the normal tasks to attend to, like keeping a job and forming relationships, that everyone has to deal with, and then there is the inner work. It's not like you get a second chance at life because you were nailing the first one. Then there's the big-picture stuff, like figuring out how we express the truth of our experience of grace through the way we live. My teachers taught me to put first things first and I did. I started with the basics, like how not to get by on fear and anger. I discovered the practices of being and the gentle world that has formed around them, and at first I felt a strong desire to leave the world of the sun behind entirely and become a child of the moon.

The problem was that I was not a child. In fact, I had been trained to be a leader and was drawn to the challenges of leadership. I knew that my healing was only just beginning, so I had to take small forays into the sun. I took a couple of volunteer positions, I went back to school, and I worked hard to become a shift leader at a restaurant. I was learning to look toward the sun without losing touch with the earth beneath my feet. The earth was my home, the moonlight my heart's rest, but the sun was my calling. I arrived at a way to grow into myself. I would point my life in the direction of my heart's desires but my focus would be on the day-to-day. Some days would be dedicated to the sun and others would be spent in silent moonlight. The moon made the sun possible and the sun gave voice to the moon. I was content to let the sun and the moon choose my path together.

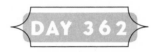

Spring comes and the grass grows all by itself.

Buddhist saying

Each of us is like a streambed where the stream is life itself. The water flows across us, expressing the unique features of our character and the life that we have lived. The sound of my life is the way the water flows across my pain and my joy, my mistakes and my willingness to learn from them. I cannot express anything else. Not knowing, and the suffering this causes, has created much of the character of my particular stream. The fear and dread that dominated my outlook growing up gave me an extremely distorted understanding of life. My work as an adult has been to discover how one forms a clear picture of the world and how to choose wisely using the information that picture provides. A lot of that work has been figuring out the extent of my ignorance. What do I think I know that I do not know?

Of the many forms of ignorance I have suffered from, the one that has pained me the most is the belief that I was alone, that I had to live my life all by myself. This is the power of touching the earth in my life. When I touch the earth in this body, this breath, this moment, I am relieved of the worst form of ignorance and I remember the bliss of being. The experience of being brings us back into the effortless manner in which everything happens, the effortless manner in which life brings us everything we need for this human adventure, the effortless manner in which spring comes and the grass grows all by itself.

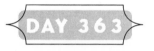

The great way is easy but people prefer the side paths.

Lao-tzu

I sat to meditate this morning knowing that later today I would finish writing this book. I moved into stillness and let myself soften into the morning around me. I felt the great way. Then my mind began to contract around what I wanted and what I did not want. I found myself a little upset about how I didn't like the way someone I knew was acting and how things are. I could feel the utter falsehood and ignorance of the stories I was telling myself. These fictions are the side paths that lure our attention away from the experience of the truth. I smiled a little at the perfect nature of the practice of yoga. Wandering down the side paths and returning to the great way over and over again, I could feel that I was getting a little better at it. A little less enamored of the side paths, a little more at home on the great way. I saw how intention takes this work and directs it. I saw how being practices train us to be responsible for the path our attention travels and how intention takes that ability and uses it in the service of our highest good.

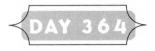
INTENTION AND BEING

Human Kindness

On May 21, 1990, I prayed for relief from suffering and I got it. My extreme obsession with alcohol was lifted and has never returned. I did not see a white light or a spectral being; I just knew that everything was going to be okay. And it has been. What I felt from the power that relieved me of the desire to drink was kindness, a powerful kindness directed at me that completely changed my place in the world. Enough kindness can make us forget ourselves and devote our lives to the service of others. I experienced that type of kindness.

In the days that followed, I observed people offering the same sort of kindness to one another all the time. To my astonishment, it became clear to me that we have the power to offer life-healing kindness to one another with no more effort than it takes us to say "Thank you" or "How are you today?" The kindness I was seeing had been there all along, I just had not had eyes to see it. I do now. I have seen the kindness in hospitals and treatment centers. I have seen the kindness in schools and sacred spaces. I have seen the kindness of mothers, fathers, and grandparents. When I am in my right mind, the kindness in my world is all I have eyes for. It is my heart's desire that we might understand the nature of human kindness, what it represents, and the world it can create, and that we might have eyes to see the kindness in our world.

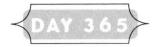

Letting Go

As a teacher, I am in the business of making statements that I hope will be helpful. I have very little time and I will never say it all; I must be content with what the moment brings, to play my part in things and to act as if I trust the process of living. This takes the courage and honesty my teachers have helped me to find. At the end of my last book, there was a lot of pain because I felt that by the time I knew what I wanted to say, the book had been written. Letting go at the end of that book was a true leap of faith. It taught me that you cannot create without being willing to let go.

Since then I have discovered that you cannot give someone something without letting go of it. When I train teachers I am giving them the training; what they do with it is up to them. I cannot make them use it in any specific way. I simply teach them and then let go, no strings attached. When I offered my wife, Mariam, my love, that is what was offered, no strings attached. When I give my children permission to choose, that is what they have been given, no strings attached. When I offer my friendship, that is what I am offering, no strings attached. For a teaching to be helpful I must say what I can say, in the time that I have, and then step back and let go.

CHAPTER SEVEN

May you be safe, may you be healthy, may you be happy, may you find your freedom, may you know peace, and may you walk through the world with ease.

Namaste.
Rolf

THREE WAYS TO EXPRESS INTENTION AND BEING

1) Aim your practice at the felt experience of the bliss of being with such regularity that you carry this experience with you as you move through your days.
2) Write down a list of your heart's desires and reflect on them often.
3) A bird flies because it knows when to flap and when to soar. The practice of yoga is knowing when to lead with being, when to lead with intention, and that one cannot exist without the other.

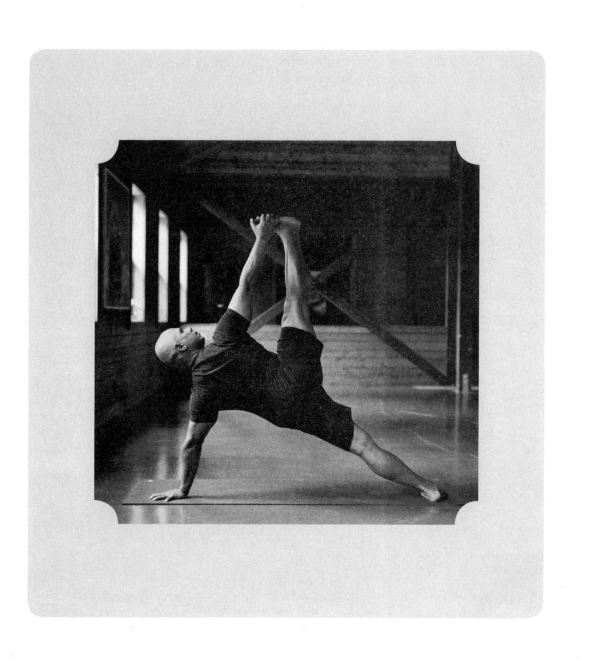

ABOUT THE AUTHOR

Rolf Gates, author of the acclaimed book on yogic philosophy *Meditations from the Mat: Daily Reflections on the Path of Yoga*, conducts yoga workshops, retreats, teacher trainings, and coaching and mentorship programs throughout the U.S. and abroad—and online. Rolf and his work have been featured in numerous media, including *Yoga Journal, ORIGINS, Natural Health, People,* and *Travel and Leisure*'s "25 Top Yoga Studios Around the World." Rolf is also the co-founder of the Yoga, Meditation and Recovery Conference at the Esalen Institute in Big Sur, California, and the Kripalu Center for Yoga & Health in Lenox, Massachusetts, as well as a teacher at Spirit Rock Meditation Center in Northern California. He is also on the advisory board for the Yoga Service Council and the Veterans Yoga Project. A former addictions counselor and U.S. Army Airborne Ranger who has practiced meditation for more than twenty-five years, Rolf brings his eclectic background to his practice and his teachings. Rolf and his wife, Mariam Gates, author of *Good Night Yoga: A Pose-by-Pose Bedtime Story,* live in Santa Cruz, California, with their two children.